Then
Comes Baby

Then Comes Baby

An Honest Conversation about Birth, Postpartum, and the Complex Transition to Parenthood

Jessica Vernon

ROWMAN & LITTLEFIELD
Lanham • Boulder • New York • London

Rowman & Littlefield
Bloomsbury Publishing Inc, 1385 Broadway, New York, NY 10018, USA
Bloomsbury Publishing Plc, 50 Bedford Square, London, WC1B 3DP, UK
Bloomsbury Publishing Ireland, 29 Earlsfort Terrace, Dublin 2, D02 AY28, Ireland
www.rowman.com

86-90 Paul Street, London EC2A 4NE, United Kingdom

Distributed by NATIONAL BOOK NETWORK

British Library Cataloguing in Publication Information Available

Library of Congress Cataloging-in-Publication Data Available

ISBN 978-1-5381-9592-5 (paperback) | ISBN 978-1-5381-9593-2 (ebook)

For product safety related questions contact productsafety@bloomsbury.com.

∞™ The paper used in this publication meets the minimum requirements of
American National Standard for Information Sciences—Permanence of Paper for
Printed Library Materials, ANSI/NISO Z39.48-1992.

For Cahya and Lyla,
the catalyst and conclusion,
this book exists because of you

CONTENTS

INTRODUCTION

When I am covering labor and delivery, part of my job is to round on—or evaluate and examine—postpartum patients who had cesarean births. During one of these days on labor and delivery, I was heading to the postpartum floor to round while amid a self-reckoning. I was in the early stages of writing this book, extremely overwhelmed with everything I was trying to do at the same time in my own life, and in panic mode, questioning if I truly had the capacity to submit the manuscript on time. I paused my own perseverating thoughts and went in to see my first patient. She was postoperative day one, meaning she had just birthed her baby via cesarean section the day prior. I put a smile on my face and introduced myself, kneeling beside her bed so that I was at eye level. Before I even asked her how she was feeling, I knew things were not going well for her. She was trying to hold it all together, but I saw the struggle in her eyes and in the tension she was holding in her body. Tears pooled in the corners of her eyes before I could even ask her how she was feeling. I stood up, grabbed some tissues, and then sat next to her as she poured out everything that had transpired in the last forty-eight hours.

She had a routine prenatal visit at thirty-nine weeks of pregnancy and was told her blood pressure was elevated and an induction of labor was recommended. She had desired spontaneous labor with minimal interventions and was hoping to labor without anesthesia. She had paused to take in what her midwife was telling her—for the safety of her and her baby, it was recommended that she toss out the old plan and go to labor and delivery directly from the office. After taking time to process, she headed to labor and delivery to meet her baby. Two days later, after a long induction of labor, a diagnosis of preeclampsia, an urgent cesarean section, a hemorrhage in the operating room, difficulty initiating breastfeeding while trying to stay coherent after no sleep, surgery, and being placed on high doses of magnesium to prevent eclamptic seizures, she was trying desperately to figure out how things had gone so drastically off course.

I sat with her for the next hour as she told her story. She needed to talk about it. She needed space and someone to be the container to hold it so she could understand what had just happened. She was desperate for someone to help her make sense of it, as she no longer recognized herself. She was not the same person who had walked into the office for her prenatal visit a few days prior. She was traumatized from her experience and couldn't look at herself in the mirror, as she did not understand the person staring back at her. She could barely look at her baby, as the baby brought back the whole experience, re-traumatizing her. This in turn made her feel so guilty because she could not bond with her baby in the way she had anticipated. She felt like she had barely started, and she was already failing at motherhood. So she cried as I held space for her, validated her feelings, and took the first steps to help her create a plan for her physical, mental, and emotional recovery.

When I left her room, I knew without a doubt that I would finish writing this book. I would write it for her and for myself and for everyone else I have cared for and met along the way who has struggled with the transition to parenthood. I know I cannot prevent all of the traumas and struggles that occur during birth and the early postpartum period. But I can share with you the knowledge and insight I have gathered over the past fifteen years that I have been caring for people during their reproductive journeys so that hopefully you do not feel like a failure or as if you are the only one going through these experiences. This does not mean I want you to give up on having a voice, asking questions, and making sure you are seen and heard and given person-centered care. I wish every birth person could have the most beautiful birth experience of their dreams and start the next chapter of their lives filled with joy and love. But I also know that we have very little control over anything in life, and as hard as that is to accept, I want you to go through this major transition understanding the realities of giving birth and caring for yourself postpartum.

The problem is society has sold us a fairy tale. Not only that, it told us exactly how each aspect of that fairy tale should look and feel. First comes love, second comes marriage, then comes the baby. So much pressure and such high expectations are placed on doing it all the "right" way, with little grace for those who cannot make it happen exactly as prescribed. If anything goes off course—something unplanned or unexpected disrupts the dream—often the birth parent feels like a failure. Something is wrong with them. Their body is broken. They were just not meant to be a parent. Because it's so much easier for everyone else, right?

All of this despite the fact that, as I mentioned earlier, so much of it is ultimately out of our control. Of those things in our control, we are all free to make different decisions on what is right for our bodies, our minds, and our families. How we should give birth, how we should recover from birth, how we should feed our baby, and how we should feel about it all are topics that can spark heated conversation and big emotional responses. Why is our ego—our identity as a parent—so tied to being able to do things in a certain way, especially when the reality is we have very limited control over any of it? And why do we stay silent about the aspects of our own experiences that do not align with how we were told it should be?

I am Dr. Jessica Vernon, an OB/GYN with a passion for holistic care and perinatal mental health care. I am also a mom of two little humans. I have provided physical, mental, and emotional support for thousands of people throughout their fertility, pregnancy, birth, and postpartum journeys and have heard countless versions of the same stories. Feelings of guilt, shame, and failure. They failed their baby. Their bodies failed them. Why is it so hard for them and so easy for everyone else? Perhaps they were never meant to be a parent. The isolation that comes from feeling so alone in your thoughts and experiences only exacerbates the problem.

I want to help you feel more prepared and less alone on your journey, so that if your experience does not align with how society told you it should be, you understand that this does not make you a failure. It makes you human. And giving birth as a human is *hard*. Becoming a parent is *hard*. I have spent so much of my time holding space and validating the feelings of birthing people who are struggling, but doing this one-on-one is not enough. I want this book to be a safe space to go where you feel less alone and more supported on your journey. Because although people give birth and become parents every day, it's not easy. Especially when you are not prepared. My hope is that by the end of this book you will feel much more knowledgeable, empowered, and prepared for your entry into parenthood so that if your story does not align with how you envisioned it or with what other people have told you it should look and feel like, you understand that you are not alone. And you have the resources and support to get through it.

DIVERSITY OF EXPERIENCE

I cannot talk about giving birth in the United States without acknowledging that I bring a lens to this not just as an OB and a mother, but also in every other aspect of who I am, starting with the fact that I have the privilege associated with my socioeconomic status as a white middle-class female. I have had access to the resources available to those with good health insurance, decent maternity leave, and financial stability. Although the physical and emotional experiences that I describe in this book are very common—and I went through many of these experiences myself even with all of my available resources and privileges—your individual experiences and perception of those experiences will undoubtedly be affected by your own identity, resources, and lived experience.

I could try to draw attention to this fact in the many chapters of this book; however, even that would be a disservice: drawing attention to certain aspects of health inequities of different marginalized communities, I could not acknowledge all of the multiple and intersectional experiences of each individual person while putting some people into large boxes such as BIPOC, AAPI, and LGBTQ+. These large boxes are all that we have, and they are still not adequate in understanding each individual person's experience. In my own practice, I try to create space for my patients to tell me about their lived experience, believe what they tell me, and make sure that they feel seen, heard, and that we are making a person-centered plan for their care. I must always acknowledge that implicit biases exist inside of me and do my best to provide care with cultural humility. My advice and recommendations are shared with my patients, but I also ask each individual patient how I can best support them. My patients honor me by sharing parts of their lives they may not share with anyone else. I cannot begin to understand my role in their healing until we make that plan together.

I also humbly accept that many of my patients may never trust me. I understand and accept that due to systemic and structural racism and as a white provider in a healthcare system that has historically mistreated and abused marginalized people, I cannot expect to be trusted by everyone. I also fully acknowledge that health equity is still a dream in most regards and that in my field, especially the state where I reside, there is a gap in maternal morbidity and mortality between white cisgender hetero birthing people and other populations, especially between white and Black birthing people. I have had many patients come into pregnancy fearing that they will not make it out alive to meet their baby. This is a real and legitimate fear, and as a white person with good health insurance giving birth in the United States, I have had the privilege to not face that fear during my pregnancies. And so, yes, I fully acknowledge that I will not be able to speak to everyone as an individual and address the systemic and institutional racism and injustices for so many marginalized communities and peoples in this book. It's too important, too vast a topic to condense into one small chapter or sprinkle throughout this book.

That said, I do my best to honor the different experiences of patients and readers through the stories and advice I share. Although every individual faces different struggles based on their experiences of pregnancy, giving birth, and becoming new parents, I believe we can find commonality and connection among those who have experienced it. I have found more common humanity in the parenthood journeys of those with extremely different life stories and backgrounds than among anyone else. I can only hope that readers feel empowered to find providers and a support system that they do trust, that treats them as individuals, and that sees and hears them. In this book, I incorporate some recommendations and support resources that I know are not available to everyone either due to location availability or to financial costs. However, I also present trusted resources throughout the chapters and at the end of the book that are free and easily accessible.

Inevitably, I am unable to cover every birthing experience. I have focused on what birth and postpartum look like with a full-term, healthy baby. If your baby is in the NICU due to prematurity or other complications, this adds another layer to your experience. I include some resources at the end for NICU parents, as this is such an important topic, but being a NICU parent is a topic that deserves its own book. If you yourself suffer from a rare, extreme complication during labor, birth, or postpartum, these topics may not be explicitly covered here. Edge cases are important and can be very scary and traumatizing. I have worked in high-volume, high-acuity hospitals for most of my career and unfortunately have seen birthing people in the ICU for many different reasons or with postpartum complications requiring further medical and surgical interventions; however, again, this is beyond the scope of this book. Regardless, I do hope that the resources I share are helpful if you or a loved one experiences one of these events, as it often takes a lot of time and processing to recover emotionally, even when you have physically healed from a serious birth complication.

HOW THIS BOOK IS ORGANIZED

The first part of the book is focused on labor, birth, and the immediate postpartum hospital stay. Giving birth in a hospital is different from a home birth or birth center birth, although there are some common threads no matter what your experience. And remember, even if you do plan on giving birth outside of a hospital, there is always a chance that your midwife may recommend transfer to a hospital facility, so knowing what that looks like is still important. I cover both spontaneous and induced labor, vaginal birth and cesarean birth, as well as what happens after the baby is out and the post-birth hospital stay until you are discharged home (hopefully with baby, occasionally not if your baby is in the NICU).

The second part of the book is focused on the early postpartum period: physical recovery, feeding your baby, emotional and mental health postpartum, as well as topics about which I commonly get questions and for which I see a lot of pressure on new parents, including exercise and sex after baby. Some of these topics are beyond my basic knowledge, so I have invited some wonderful experts to add more depth and wisdom to this section. In conversation with them, I experienced many moments in which I learned something so helpful that I wish I had known it when I was going through my postpartum journey, and I have incorporated a lot of it here for you.

Part III focuses on the myths of motherhood, the importance of community, and self-care. This book is about *you*, not your baby. I love babies. I love my babies. But I also have come to learn that I am the most important person in their lives, and if I am not healthy, happy, and thriving, it affects my kids, my family, and my community. So I want to reframe how we view ourselves and how we view each other as parents. If we don't put ourselves first, who will? If we don't show society our value and how new parents should be supported, who will? I don't have all of the answers, but I do know that reframing how I view my role and identity as a parent and rejecting the judgment and criticism of others, as well as my own self-criticism, has enabled me to thrive in ways I never had before. And I hope to instill a sense of this in you as well, because you deserve it.

As we start this journey, I want to delve into the idea of a perfect birth, birth plans, and why certain things may be required per hospital policy or recommended by your provider that may go against the preferences set forth in your birth plan. And ultimately, I want to look at the big picture and your top priorities and biggest goals, as this may ultimately not align with certain aspects of your birth plan. I am so excited to go on this journey with you, to show you a little bit of the world I have been living in for most of my adult life, and what I have learned from my experiences as well as those of all of my most incredible teachers—my patients.

PART I

Labor and Birth

ONE

THERE IS NO ONE RIGHT WAY
TO GIVE BIRTH

I once heard a hospital consultant say that labor and delivery is a cross between a wedding and an emergency room. Just like on a wedding day, you might have a vision for how things will go in a perfect, idealized state, but often things do not go according to plan. It can be disappointing if you are not prepared for all of the possible ways and reasons your birth experience may not reflect what you envisioned. The truth is this: there's no right way to give birth; there are only preferences. If you do make a birth plan, make a plan that is flexible and give yourself compassion when things don't go as planned. Sometimes this means small changes, such as birth parents deciding they want an epidural, or big changes, such as needing an emergency C-section. I have seen many birth parents so set on accomplishing their ideal birth goals that when things do not go according to plan, they feel like failures as parents and as people whose bodies are supposed to "intuitively know what to do." I always try to help my patients truly believe that every birth is sacred in its own right, no matter how it happens. The goal is a safe and healthy baby and birth parent.

I have cared for countless patients who have needed cesarean births after days of labor when it becomes clear that their babies are not fitting through their pelvises for one reason or another. Often these conversations are very difficult, because they really wanted a vaginal birth and often never even had prepared for the possibility of a C-section. These conversations usually involve a lot of tears and require time to process this unexpected reality. After the surgery, some parents meet their babies and are so grateful that they and their babies came out on the other side healthy that they come to peace with the fact that they needed a C-section. Others do not cope as well with the change in plans and occasionally even comment that it was the worst day of their lives. My hope is that every birth parent would feel safe and prepared for whatever reality awaits them on one of the most important, precious days of their lives.

Every doctor wants to respect and honor the birth parent's preferences, but sometimes we have to take action to ensure a safe and healthy delivery—even if that means disappointing the birth parent. Maternal deaths and stillbirths do occur in the United States at a higher rate than is acceptable, although the situation is much more dire in many parts of the developing world that do not have ready access to modern medicine and hospitals. In the developing world, the rate of birth injuries to the mother and baby are also much higher. Babies may survive but have permanent brain injury. Mothers may endure traumatic birth injuries, such as fistulas, and be exiled from their communities. Every time I take lifesaving action in the delivery room, I'm grateful that we have resources and procedures to protect the lives of birth parents and babies who may not otherwise fare well.

I once met a patient who had recently come to the United States from a rural part of the developing world. She had a placenta previa (placenta covering the cervix) in her current pregnancy and would need a C-section birth. I thought initially she would be scared of the C-section, as her other births had been vaginal. When I spoke to her, she told me that at home where she birthed her other children, there were no blood products available in the hospital, so a patient would need to bring blood with them if a transfusion was anticipated. She was extremely scared about the increased risk of hemorrhage during her delivery, which from her lived experience meant a high risk of dying if she lost too much blood. She was so surprised and comforted to realize that this was not the case in the hospital where she would give birth this time. Due to our access to a blood bank and medications to help decrease bleeding, her risk of severe injury or death from massive blood loss was extremely low. Encounters like this one have helped me reframe birth and make space for all of the surprises that occurred during my own labor and birth.

Birth experiences are often shared and publicized across social media. In the best cases, this celebration of birth has helped many women overcome their fears and feel empowered. But it can also lead to a greater sense of judgment and loneliness if you feel your birth experience differs from what you see online. There are images all over social media of women having unmedicated home births, often referred to as "natural births," as if giving birth any other way is not natural. These birth stories are wonderful, but they are only one type of birth story. The idealized images run the risk of making you feel that if you are unable to achieve an unmedicated birth or even a vaginal birth, you are a failure.

The truth is that all births can be empowering and beautiful. I was extremely humbled during labor with my first daughter. I had such intense back pain with my contractions that I asked for pain medication when I was only two centimeters dilated. I definitely felt that I must be weak because I could not tolerate the contractions when I was not even in active labor. I never did get into active labor and I share more of my birth story later—however, I will say I was extremely grateful for morphine sedation and my epidural, even though my initial goal (due mostly to the fact that I wanted to prove myself capable in a society where this was idealized, not because it was actually a personal imperative) was to have an unmedicated birth.

I often see patients who come into the office or to labor and delivery with very detailed birth plans. It's hard to articulate to someone I have just met that although I'll try my best to do everything the way they envision, expectations often don't meet reality. I don't want to come across as one of those doctors who will move quickly toward interventions, effectively taking away the birth person's autonomy, so unless I have already gained the patient's trust, I do not voice everything that I am thinking. So here

There is a good chance your labor and birth will not go exactly as you have envisioned. That doesn't mean it can't be good.

it is, unfiltered and honest: there is a good chance your labor and birth will not go exactly as you have envisioned. That doesn't mean it can't be good.

BIRTH PLANS ARE REALLY BIRTH PREFERENCES

Birth plans, which I prefer to call "birth preferences" or "birth wishes," are comprehensive documents stating how the birth parent prefers to give birth. There are countless examples of birth plans online, and your care provider or hospital may also have sample documents for you to use. The amount of detail and focus on specific areas of the experience varies among different birth plans. I do not have a particular birth plan template that I love, so I recommend looking at a few to familiarize yourself with them and then asking your provider about any language in the plan that you do not understand. A patient once brought me a birth plan and had checked all of the aspects that she had heard an influencer on Instagram say she should check, including a lotus birth, which neither of us even understood. When I googled it, I saw that it meant keeping the placenta attached to the baby for weeks after birth until the umbilical cord shriveled and detached. Once I explained this to the patient, she immediately told me she definitely did *not* want that and would prefer to go home with her baby without afterbirth in tow.

All birth plans include details regarding the ambiance while laboring and giving birth, such as who will be in the room, how you prefer the birthing environment, if you want pain control during labor and birth, what type of labor augmentation and interventions you are okay with and which you want to avoid, immediate care of your baby after birth, and whether or not you would like to breastfeed/chestfeed. Birth plans are wonderful in that they can empower you to think about your goals and priorities as well as decrease your anxiety around your birth experience before it happens. It can help the care team to provide person-centered care. However, they can also lead to expectations that often do not match reality. Just remember that ultimately there's no right way to give birth, and there is no way to completely control your birth process, so create a birth plan that leaves room for flexibility and surprises, rank the importance of the elements of your birth plan, and give yourself compassion when things don't go as planned.

Although it's wonderful to have an idea about how you want to birth your baby, the perfect birth cannot be planned. Plus, there are many circumstances under which your goals and preferences may change. Being too rigid in your plans makes it harder for you to negotiate these changes with yourself and your support team. Incorporate some flexibility in your birth plan to allow for the unknown. And develop self-compassion around your body and your birth so that if things go off course, you do not see it as a failure.

WHAT YOUR DOCTOR WANTS YOU
TO KNOW ABOUT YOUR BIRTH PLAN

You probably have a birth plan, even if it is not a physical document but an ideal version of birth in your mind. I want you to feel empowered to envision an ideal birth where you feel comfortable and centered in your birth experience, but I also want you to accept and be prepared for the fact that many things are ultimately not in our control and often things do not go according to plan but that does not mean you can't have a beautiful birth.

When I spoke to Kelsey Power, a licensed clinical psychologist and reproductive mental health specialist who specializes in trauma and the perinatal period, she shared the following lens on birth plans with me:

> I relate to [the birth plan] both as a metaphor for how you're thinking about this experience and as an actual concrete birth plan. In the metaphor, you are telling me about your relationship to feeling out of control or in control and your own sense of power or disempowerment. I really am pretty explicit that being rigid is going to set you up for more distress because [birth] is unpredictable and there's a balance between being educated and knowledgeable about your preferences, which is super important, and [the fact] that you have very little control over what ends up happening. Being able to sit with that and how hard that is to know, think about, and feel really requires some flexibility.[1]

In the following pages, I discuss some of the topics covered in a typical birth plan in which I see the most friction occur. I want you to understand what parts of the experience should be considered the default, things you should always be able to expect from your provider and care team, as they are now considered the standard of care. I also explain the context around the variations among hospitals and how the protocols may make it more difficult in some instances to adhere to certain requests in your birth plan. I explain why doctors might deviate from what is routine, depending on the situation and risks to the birth parents and/or baby.

As an OB/GYN who has witnessed things not going according to plan for so many of my patients, my first pregnancy was the first time in life that I truly understood that I had no control over what happened. It was scary and uncomfortable to sit with that and I tried to avoid acknowledging the fact as much as possible. As Dr. Power states, "I think there tends to be an over-promise of what control we have in the vein of being educated, which is obviously, crucially important. But I think we mislead people. And maybe we mislead ourselves with the wish of being able to have something a certain way."

In this book, I don't want to mislead you. I don't want to make false promises. I know that you can be extremely prepared and educated and "do everything right" during your pregnancy, and still things often do not go according to plan during birth and the early postpartum period. You might also unexpectedly decide to change your plan. None of these changes makes you, or your body, a failure. So let's make sure you are not just educated about your options, but also understand why flexibility might be necessary for your and your baby's health.

Some birth plans may include a lot of personal preferences, such as factors that influence the mood in the labor room (lighting, music, clothing preferences, etc.), how and if you will be given instructions during pushing, and if you want to collect cord blood or keep the placenta. These are all personal decisions that may change your experience, but from a clinical standpoint, they do not make a difference in your outcomes and will generally not be affected by any complications during labor or birth, so I will not comment on them here.

No matter what, it is very important to know that no one should ever do anything to you without first asking permission. Before any procedure, your medical team should fully explain the risks, benefits, and alternatives so that you feel that you understand and are part of the decision-making process. Of course, some situations are emergencies, and things may happen very quickly, but if you have thought about all of the possibilities and have built trust and understanding with your care team, even emergencies can happen without causing trauma in their aftermath. It is not the specific situation, but how it is perceived by the person experiencing it that determines if it becomes traumatic or even leads to post-traumatic stress disorder.

Keep in mind that many elements of a birth plan apply only to those who plan to give birth in a hospital setting. A home birth or a birth at an outpatient birth center will eliminate some of the options available at a hospital but may offer others that are not available. Below I cover some of the aspects of common birth plans that tend to cause the most friction and distress when experience or provider recommendations vary from your preferences and expectations. I address them in order of how they often are encountered upon entering the hospital. Please remember that if your providers make a recommendation, it is not because they are trying to take away your autonomy or medicalize your experience; it is for your and your baby's safety. Once you are at the hospital and these topics come up, it can be hard for providers to suggest interventions and for you to trust our motivation. Thinking about these things and having conversations with your care team in advance can be helpful in reframing your goals and expectations.

Intravenous (IV) Access

Intravenous (IV) access is mandatory in most hospitals as a cautionary measure. It does not mean that you must have fluids running through the IV or be tied to an IV pole. However, if your labor is being induced or augmented with Pitocin (a medication used to induce or augment labor and to help the uterus contract after labor—more on why this may be recommended later), you will need IV fluids. If you are getting a cesarean section, you will need IV fluids, as well as if you are getting an epidural, as it is important to get a lot of fluids prior to epidural placement to avoid a drop in your blood pressure.

Even if you would like to decline fluids, hospitals still encourage you to have an IV placed. In an emergency such as a hemorrhage (excessive bleeding), an emergency cesarean delivery, or the need for emergency IV medications, the team does not waste precious time trying to start an IV instead of taking care of you and your baby. That said, you always have the right to refuse any intervention, if you are aware of the risks. If I have a patient in spontaneous labor, whose baby's heart rate is reassuring, who is not anemic at baseline and does not have a high risk of hemorrhage, and who prefers to avoid IV placement, I think it is reasonable to decline the IV, as long as the patient understand the risks in an emergency. I work with the team at the hospital to help such patients achieve their goals. Pitocin is also typically given by IV after any delivery to help the uterus contract and prevent hemorrhage, but this medication can also be given as an intramuscular injection (a shot in the muscle, typically the thigh) if you prefer. Again, I think it is reasonable to decline the Pitocin if you understand the risks of hemorrhage and are at low risk for bleeding. We always have medications to help control bleeding available in the hospital if they become necessary.

Fetal Monitoring

Monitoring of the baby's heart rate may be continuous or intermittent. Intermittent monitoring protocol varies from hospital to hospital: checking the heartbeat hourly during labor after an initial twenty-minute period of reassuring tracing followed by intermittent or continuous monitoring once the birth parent starts to push. You may prefer intermittent monitoring so that you're free to move around, especially if wireless monitoring is not an option (continuous monitors that do not need to be plugged into a machine). There are exceptions to being a candidate for intermittent fetal monitoring: The birth parent must not be receiving any medication for induction or augmentation of labor. They also cannot be on any medication such as magnesium, a medication used in people who develop very high blood pressures and/or other symptoms of preeclampsia. This is a good question to ask your care team in advance so you understand the options at the hospital where you will give birth and the restrictions regarding intermittent monitoring, if that is one of your goals.

Pain Relief

Depending on the hospital where you give birth, you may have different options available for medicated pain relief. I discuss the various medicated pain management options further in a later chapter. Pain management tends to be a major area in which expectations differ from experience. It is very common for birthing parents to desire an unmedicated birth; however, if you change your mind during labor and request pain management, you are not a failure. Your labor course and the pain you experience can vary greatly depending on how many babies you have had before, the size and position of your baby, the shape of your body, your genetic makeup in regard to pain tolerance and how quickly your body labors, whether your water breaks early in labor or before labor, and if you are induced or your labor is augmented in any way. I always recommend at least understanding the options available at your hospital and the risks and benefits of each before the birthday or hospital admission. Once you are in labor, you may be in so much pain that it is hard to focus and understand everything the anesthesiologist tells you at that point.

Induction of Labor

Induction of labor may be recommended for many reasons. The most common reason is that you are past your due date and getting closer to the forty-two-week mark when stillbirth rates increase. For older birth parents, providers sometimes recommend induction closer to the due date as opposed to waiting until forty-one weeks; however, there is no definitive recommendation from the American College of Obstetricians and Gynecologists on the exact timing of post-date (after the due date) induction if the pregnancy is uncomplicated. I share more details regarding induction of labor in chapter 3.

Labor and Birth Positions

As long as the baby's heart rate can be monitored and is reassuring and you are not receiving pain medication that requires you to sit or lie down to avoid falling, then you should be able to move around during labor and get into any comfortable position.

This also applies to birthing positions. There are many birthing positions that are more physiologic and feel more natural when pushing, especially when the birthing person does not have an epidural. Certain positions, such as squatting or being on your hands and knees, actually open up the pelvis more than lying flat on your back with legs in stirrups (called dorsal lithotomy). There are caveats, however, and this is definitely something to discuss with your delivering provider prior to your baby's birthday. Many physicians were not taught how to deliver in other positions, so they are uncomfortable delivering babies in anything other than dorsal lithotomy. If your doctor is uncomfortable with you giving birth in other positions on the day of and there is not a medical indication, you can always ask if there is another provider available who is more flexible. Or you can try to negotiate with your doctor so that you can modify the position in ways that make it more comfortable to you—not lowering your head as much, for instance, or not breaking the bed down (taking the bottom off of the bed) so that you can rest your legs on the bed in between pushes. If the baby's heart rate is not reassuring near the end of pushing, your doctor may recommend dorsal lithotomy so that an episiotomy or operative delivery can be conducted if necessary. These lifesaving procedures cannot be safely performed from other positions.

Episiotomies

An episiotomy is a cut made at the opening of the vagina to make more room for the baby. Many years ago, episiotomies were a routine practice, as it was thought that making a cut on the perineum would create a wound that healed better than with natural tearing. However, subsequent studies have shown this is not true and that when the perineum tears naturally, it heals better. Therefore, the current standard of care is not to perform an episiotomy unless necessary, and if the provider thinks it is necessary, they must get permission from the patient first. Reasons why an episiotomy may be recommended include:

1. The baby's heart rate is not reassuring, but the baby is close to delivering vaginally and an episiotomy will expedite delivery.

2. The birthing person is exhausted and does not have energy to continue to push but is close to a vaginal delivery. In this case, an episiotomy will expedite delivery without the need for an operative delivery with vacuum or forceps.
3. To avoid a tear into the rectum if an operative delivery is needed.
4. A shoulder dystocia: the baby's head delivers and the shoulder gets stuck behind the birth parent's pubic bone, necessitating additional maneuvers to safely deliver the baby. If one of the maneuvers performed involves putting the provider's hand into the patient's vagina to help release the arm or rotate the baby, sometimes an episiotomy is needed to make enough space to accommodate the provider's hand.

In all of these instances, there is a reason that a provider performs an episiotomy other than simply expediting delivery. There must be a maternal or fetal indication, and the birthing person must be aware of and agree to the procedure.

Just like tearing, an episiotomy is painful if you do not have a good epidural or local anesthetic. If the doctor is going to cut an episiotomy, they should always inject local anesthesia first for pain control, unless they have tested that you are numb from your epidural. Even if I do not have the prior delivery notes of a patient in labor, I can usually tell if they have had an episiotomy from the thin white scar and let them know in advance that that previous scar tissue is weaker and more likely to separate during the birth than a perineal tear that has occurred naturally.

Operative Delivery

Similar to the episiotomy, a vacuum or forceps should be applied only if there is a maternal or fetal indication; the provider has explained the risks, benefits, and alternatives; and the birth person has agreed to the procedure. Here are the reasons your doctor might recommend an operative delivery:

1. If the baby's heart rate is not reassuring, delivery needs to be expedited, and the baby is low enough to be delivered with a

vacuum or forceps but not low enough to deliver easily with only an episiotomy.

2. If the birthing person is exhausted and cannot push anymore and the baby is low enough.

Depending on the provider's training, comfort level, and the position of the baby, they may offer the option of a vacuum, forceps, or both. The art of forceps-assisted delivery is not often mastered in residency now, so many more operative deliveries are performed via vacuum than with forceps. This is something you can discuss with your provider prior to the birthday. Only physicians perform operative deliveries, and they are only performed in the hospital. If you are in the care of a midwife, they may need to transfer your care to a physician if vacuum or forceps are recommended. In any of these instances, if the baby is too high or the head is rotated in such a way that the provider feels it is not safe to perform an operative delivery, the only option may be a cesarean birth.

Patients might also choose a cesarean birth (C-section) if they do not want to accept the risks of the vacuum or forceps to help deliver the baby vaginally. The risks of a vacuum delivery include scalp bruises and abrasions, petechiae (broken blood vessels) in the baby's eyes, and—very rare but more severe—bleeding inside the baby's brain. Also, if there is a failed vacuum (i.e., the baby does not deliver with normal traction on the vacuum while the birth person is pushing or the vacuum pops off/loses suction from the baby's head too many times), then the only alternative is a C-section. A C-section after a failed vacuum can be worse, as the baby may be wedged into the pelvis, making it difficult to deliver the head and a greater risk of bleeding and damage to the uterus and bladder during delivery. The use of forceps also risks scalp bruising and lacerations; if applied incorrectly or with too much force, it can also lead to damage to the baby's skull bones and bleeding in the baby's brain. Any operative delivery has an increased risk of third and fourth degree perineal lacerations, or tears into the rectum, which is why the provider often recommends an episiotomy that angles the tear away from the rectum (called a mediolateral episiotomy). These complications do sound really scary, and they are, which is why an operative delivery must be done under the right circumstances and by a competent physician who has fully assessed the situation and counseled the patient.

Cesarean Section

Unless there is a reason that it would be unsafe to have a vaginal birth, or the birthing person requests a primary elective C-section (for which there are multiple valid reasons), the default goal of any obstetrician is to try for a vaginal birth versus recommending a cesarean birth. Risks of a C-section include more pain and bleeding than an average vaginal birth, increased risk of infection, damage to pelvic organs such as the uterus, the bladder, and the bowels, as well as the rare risks of permanent injury or death to the birth parent and/or baby. Therefore, vaginal births have fewer inherent risks in most cases and a C-section will not be recommended without a clear indication, usually when a vaginal birth is no longer considered safe for birth parent and/or baby. I discuss cesarean birth in detail in chapter 5.

Infant Care

Depending on the hospital in which you give birth, its staffing model, and staff training, you may encounter a variety of routine practices in immediate newborn care. Hospitals that are more patient centered typically encourage delayed cord clamping for at least one minute and immediate skin-to-skin contact of the newborn with the birth parent. Basic stimulation, drying, and resuscitation of the baby can still happen while the baby remains on the birth parent, as long as other interventions are not necessary. Administration of erythromycin and vitamin K while the baby is on the birth parent may also be offered. Erythromycin is an antibiotic given as an eye ointment after birth to decrease the risk of chlamydia infecting the baby's eyes, which can result in blindness. Vitamin K is a shot given to the baby after birth to help the baby's blood to clot. Babies are not born with enough of this clotting factor, which can lead to serious bleeding if the clotting factor is not given.

Talk to your provider prior to the birth—at your prenatal visits if possible—to get an idea of common practices at your birthing facility. Some facilities, if their staff is overwhelmed or they have outdated practices, will take the baby immediately to the warmer for full assessment, assigning of Apgar scores, drying suction if necessary, and the administration of medications. No matter how wonderful your provider is and how often they ask staff to respect your wishes, the nurses and/or pediatricians are the ones doing the majority of the newborn care while your provider and primary nurse tend to your needs, so they may do what is most convenient or routine in their environment, even if you ask for things to be done a different way. I have attended births in many different hospital settings, and some are very patient and baby centered, whereas others are more task oriented. I have fought many battles to keep babies with moms—some I have won, some I have lost, and always with criticism from the staff I was arguing with afterward. All of this is mentioned to provide you with the opportunity to inform yourself. Ask your provider for an honest overview about what to expect in the facility where you will give birth. Rather than telling you that they will respect your birth preferences, ask your provider to tell you what to anticipate from the hospital staff. You can also ask other friends or parents who have delivered at the facility where you plan on giving birth to tell you what their experiences were like.

If you have a scheduled or unanticipated cesarean birth, please be aware that this will involve a different set of practices and procedures for infant care, as well. Delayed cord clamping may still be possible depending on how the baby looks and the amount of bleeding from the uterus at the time of birth. If the cord has to be cut to stabilize the birth parent's bleeding or the baby's respiratory status, then delayed cord clamping may not be feasible. In most hospitals, your partner or support person cannot cut the cord in order to maintain the sterility of the environment and avoid the risk of infection. Some facilities are finding creative ways to allow the support person to cut the cord at time of delivery, and others will have the support person come to the warmer to trim the cord. Every hospital I have worked in has always required the baby to be passed immediately to the pediatric team or baby nurse for assessment after a cesarean birth, as there is a higher chance of amniotic fluid aspiration when delivered via cesarean section. If this happens, the baby may have trouble breathing or even get an infection in their lungs.

My second daughter had to go to the NICU for her first forty-eight hours for oxygen support due to amniotic fluid aspiration after I gave birth via C-section. When she was gurgling and grunting in the operating room, I knew immediately that she may need some extra oxygen support to open up her lungs. Many parents are not prepared for this possibility and don't understand the importance of good suctioning of the nose and mouth on C-section babies immediately after birth. After a C-section, babies are usually taken immediately to the warmer to be given medications, so please let the nurse or pediatric team know when you get to the operating room if you are declining erythromycin and/or vitamin K, as these staff may not have been in your labor room and may be unaware of your preferences. Be prepared that in many states, these are mandatory medications, so if you decline them, you may have to sign against medical advice papers or have a longer discussion with the pediatric team. No matter what the decision, it is common to have to explain your reasoning over and over; this is simply due to strict hospital policies and laws when it comes to newborn medications and the need to follow hospital and state protocols in these situations. It is also difficult to do skin-to-skin with the birth parent immediately after a cesarean birth, and in cases when it is not possible, the support person in the room can do skin-to-skin while in the operating room, and then the baby can go skin-to-skin on the birth parent in the recovery area. More on this in a later chapter.

Feeding

Chapter 10 discusses feeding plans in more detail. All I will say here is to please have a backup plan in place if you plan to breastfeed/chestfeed and are unable to initiate feeding within the first few hours of your baby's life. Common examples of when this may occur are when your baby is in the NICU, you are not producing enough colostrum, or the baby is not able to latch effectively. This may mean stating that you are okay with formula supplementation. Hospitals have formula available to give to the babies if needed, so you do not have to bring your own. Some hospitals have donor milk, so you can ask if this is an option for you at the place you will give birth if you prefer that over formula.

PRIORITIZE WHAT MATTERS MOST TO YOU

No matter what your individual priorities and goals are, every parent that I have worked with ultimately wants a safe birth and a healthy baby. Everything else then must be prioritized and will vary depending on the person giving birth, their lived experience, personal values, and wishes. When thinking about your labor and birth experience, besides making a list of your preferences or completing a birth plan, think about how you rank each of these items. There should be one or a few things that are the most important to you and about which you are least flexible. Others may be "nice to have" but will not make or break your experience.

I wish for every birth person to feel seen, heard, and respected during their labor and birth. As with every other aspect of life, we may have the illusion of control, but the reality is far different, which is why it is so important to have self-compassion and not blame yourself when things do not go according to plan. Focusing on how you receive care, who is present, and if you feel empowered and centered during the labor and birth will be the most important factors when you look back and remember the day (or days) you spent in labor and giving birth to your baby—which are the topics of chapters 2 and 3.

TWO

SPONTANEOUS LABOR

When you envision going into labor, what does it look like? If you are like most first-time parents, you probably imagine that you are standing in your kitchen, having a nice conversation with your partner while preparing dinner together, and then, suddenly, you feel an intense pain—you just had a contraction! Then your water breaks. A huge gush of fluid comes out and onto the floor—thank goodness you were at home and not out shopping or at work! You tell your partner the baby is coming. As they rush around gathering the hospital bag, calling your parents, and putting the hospital address in the GPS, your contractions rapidly progress to intense, almost unbearable pain, and you tell your partner to hurry—you might not make it to the hospital in time. All the way to the hospital, you are screaming and grabbing their arm, scared that you will give birth in the car with your partner catching the baby. You make it to the hospital just in time to get wheeled into a room, where you push for just a few contractions, and your beautiful, pink, screaming newborn enters the world. The scene ends with the baby in your arms and your partner at your side, both of you with tears in your eyes and so in love with your new baby.

The reality is that labor can be more nuanced and complex than most first-time birth parents expect. I have had patients come to the office for a routine appointment or ultrasound, and I find out that their water broke days before. Because they did not start contracting afterward, they assumed that they peed on themselves or had extra-watery discharge. Rarely does labor happen as quickly and seamlessly as in the movies, especially if it is your first baby.

The thought of going into labor, whether spontaneous or induced, is highly anticipated and often anxiety provoking for those who know it is in their future. This is because we have all seen portrayals of labor and birth on TV, in the movies, and even in videos of labor and birth on social media, but we cannot predict how it will look or feel for us until it happens. In this chapter, I walk you through the earliest stages of spontaneous labor (going into labor naturally, without the use of medications or augmentations to prompt labor to occur) so that you know what is happening in your body and what you can expect as you progress to the hospital.

I frequently get calls from pregnant patients whose water broke but who aren't yet in labor who are having contractions that aren't regular or painful or are experiencing other symptoms that may or may not warrant coming into the hospital. I discuss which symptoms require calling your doctor and coming into labor and delivery versus when you can stay at home.

Labor is an awe-inspiring process that our bodies are uniquely equipped for.

Labor is an awe-inspiring process that our bodies are uniquely equipped for. Though there are sure to be surprises along the way, I hope that for all birth parents this is an empowering experience that shows you just how incredible your body is.

WHEN LABOR HAPPENS

Many first-time parents think they will go into labor on their due date. Due dates are estimates based on your last menstrual period and your early ultrasound or sometimes on the date of an IVF transfer; however, this in no way means that your baby will arrive on that specific date. In fact, only around 5 percent of babies decide to be born on their official due date. More likely, your baby will arrive within a couple weeks of that date.

It can be confusing to keep track of all of the terms that doctors and medical professionals use regarding the dates that you begin labor. See table 2.1 for a helpful breakdown of the terms used depending on when your labor starts. Full term is considered 37 to 41 weeks; that's the ideal. And the good news is that spontaneous labor most often occurs at full term, between 37 weeks, 0 days, and 41 weeks, 6 days. Even more commonly, we can narrow that range down to 39 to 41 weeks. Labor that happens early term (37 weeks, 0 days, to 38 weeks, 6 days) is still considered full term, but less common. If this isn't your first pregnancy and you have a history of delivering early term or going past 41 weeks, history often repeats itself, so you can anticipate it may happen again.

Labor that occurs spontaneously prior to 37 weeks is called preterm labor. If your labor starts during this period before reaching full term, your providers, with or without the consultation of high-risk specialists, may try to stop the labor, or they may deem it safer for you and/or baby to allow labor to progress and give birth, depending on the situation.

If you are still pregnant at 42 weeks, your pregnancy is considered post-term. During this period, the risk of stillbirth and other serious adverse outcomes increases significantly, so recommendations are to deliver by 42 weeks, even if that means that labor must be induced.

Table 2.1. Gestational Age Categories

Gestational Age	Terminology
20–36	preterm
37–38	(early) full term
39–40	full term
41	(late) full term
42+	post-term

WHAT HAPPENS IN LABOR

I wish all of you the labor I did not have: a nice progression through early labor, timing your hospital arrival with the onset of active labor, with your water still intact, and with time for an epidural and to get comfortable prior to the birth, if you so desire. Alas, labor is not one-size-fits-all, and there are so many factors that vary from person to person. If you take a birth class and do your research, listening to the stories of friends and relatives who have been there before, you may already be able to appreciate this fact. Even people who had babies before are often surprised when their labor course is substantially different the second, third, or fourth time. So let's cover the basics, the nuances of labor, and some factors that may contribute to differences in labor patterns and progression.

Labor is divided into three stages:

Stage 1: start of labor until you are fully dilated (10 centimeters)
Stage 2: fully dilated until the baby is born
Stage 3: birth of the baby until the placenta is out

Stages 2 and 3 are discussed in the next few chapters. Stage 1 is reviewed here, as it is important to the understanding of labor and when and why your provider may recommend augmenting labor (using the same mechanisms as for induction, but once labor has already started but is not progressing).

Stage 1: Latent and Active Labor

The first stage of labor is divided into a latent phase and an active phase. The latent phase is defined as from the start of labor until 5 centimeters of dilation, often called "early labor." The active phase is from 6 centimeters of dilation until fully dilated, or 10 centimeters dilated.

Until recently, many obstetric practitioners followed the Friedman curve, a chart that aimed to describe the average progression of labor.

The Friedman curve is based on a study published by Emanuel Friedman in 1954 that tracked the labor of five hundred white women at one hospital center in New York City and plotted their labor course.[1] Yes, that's correct—only white women were in the study, not because there were not Black and Brown birthing people in New York City at the time, but because many hospitals, including the one where Dr. Friedman worked, were segregated at the time. On average, the patients were also younger and weighed less than the average birthing person today. They also did not have epidurals, as this was a time when twilight sedation was the standard for pain control in labor, and babies were delivered by forceps about half of the time. Often, a woman was half asleep during labor, so she couldn't even understand what was happening, let alone push out her baby.

As you can see, besides the many unethical aspects of birthing during the time of Friedman's study, it is not representative of the diversity and changing characteristics of birthing people and labor practices in many ways. It never should have become the standard for determining how labor should progress. However, this was what was taught to generations of obstetricians, including me, and it was not updated until recent years.

If your doctor was following the Friedman curve, they might have concluded that your labor wasn't progressing as quickly as it should or perhaps even told you that there was "failure to progress," when in reality your body may have been progressing at its own perfectly normal pace. Unfortunately, following this outdated model has resulted in countless unnecessary C-sections throughout the years.

The good news is that doctors no longer follow the Friedman curve. The new guidelines from the American College of Obstetricians and Gynecologists (ACOG) state that a failed induction of labor (or labor that does not get into active labor) occurs when someone has had their water broken and been on Pitocin for twelve to eighteen hours without reaching 6 centimeters. An arrest of dilation can be diagnosed only in active labor, or at 6 or more centimeters of dilation.

Stage 1(a): Latent Labor

Latent labor may take a few hours or a few days. It may also start and stall many times (prodromal labor) before fully kicking in and progressing to active labor. The most common sign of labor is contractions, which initially may feel like tightening or period-like cramps. Depending on the position of the baby, you may feel contractions more in your abdomen or in your lower back, so do not dismiss the pain if it is persistent and recurrent, even if it does not feel like it is in your uterus. Typically, when contractions occur every three or four minutes for a few hours and are painful enough that you have to stop talking to breathe through them, you are making cervical change and progressing in labor. This is a good time to call your provider and let them know, if you have not already.

You may also lose your mucus plug or experience bloody show in early labor. The mucus plug is just that—a thick plug of mucus, often tinged with blood from your cervix. This plug helps protect the uterus and prevent bacteria from the vagina from getting through the cervix to the amniotic sac, or bag of water, where the baby lives. You may lose this plug prior to labor, even weeks before, if your cervix starts to thin out and open up slightly (or "ripen"). This is okay—it does not mean your baby will get an infection. Your mucus plug also may come out once you are in early labor.

You will not know how far you are dilated until you have a cervical exam; however, there are a few general signs that may help you understand when you are transitioning to active labor if you are doing the early part of labor at home. Bloody show tends to occur when your labor is transitioning from latent, or early labor, to active labor. Often, when getting close to active labor (4 or 5 centimeters dilated), the intensity of contractions increases, the baby gets lower, and the dilation leads to some spotting. If there is more bleeding, like a period, this is concerning, and you should notify your provider immediately. Some people also break their water in early labor or even before going into labor. If it happens spontaneously (meaning your provider does not artificially break your water), the water often breaks around 8 centimeters of labor. However, I have had many patients over the years whose water broke before experiencing any contractions who did not call because nothing drastic seemed to change, contrary to what they've seen depicted in the movies. Not everyone who breaks their water early in labor will feel contractions at that time, and the contractions may not even start at all without induction to get the process started.

Stage 1(b): Active Labor

Active labor typically progresses more rapidly, but this stage still varies a lot based on the birthing person, the baby's size and position, and the size and shape of the birthing person's pelvis. The strength of contractions can be measured only by an internal contraction monitor, called an intrauterine pressure catheter, and not from an external contraction monitor, or fetal tocometer. This means that as long as a birthing person continues to make progress from one exam to the next and everything is reassuring with them and the baby, doctors should no longer recommend C-sections after two hours without any cervical change (the standard during the time of the Friedman curve). ACOG guidelines define an arrest of dilation as no cervical change once in active labor with four hours of adequate or six hours of inadequate contractions. I always tell patients that if they have a bigger baby, are having their first baby after age thirty-five, or have been diagnosed with obesity or any other factor that can make labor progress slower, I already anticipate that labor may progress on the slower side, and that is totally fine.

WHEN SHOULD YOU CALL YOUR PROVIDER?

If you think you are in labor, when should you call your provider? This depends on your history and where you are giving birth, so ask your provider for any specifics. For instance, if you live in a more rural area or your doctor takes calls from home, meaning they are not in the hospital ready for anyone and everyone who may arrive in labor, then they will give you recommendations for how soon to call with symptoms. Also, if you have a history of cesarean birth, a history of fast labors, or something specific to the current pregnancy, such as a very small baby that may not tolerate labor well or a lot of amniotic fluid (called polyhydramnios) where it is safer to be in the hospital when your water breaks, then your provider may recommend you come earlier as well. Also, if at any point in early labor or in general you feel the baby is moving much less than is typical for you or is not moving at all, please call your provider and go to the hospital. When contractions start, you may feel less movement than normal when the uterus is contracting strongly, as the baby is balled up in your contracted uterus, but between contractions, the baby can resume their normal activity.

REASONS TO CALL YOUR PROVIDER

1. You have a medical or logistical reason for which your provider has told you to call as soon as you go into labor.
2. You experience painful, regular contractions that you have to breathe through (during which you are unable to talk) every three or four minutes for two or more hours. If contractions space out with rest and hydration, you are in prodromal labor or false labor.
3. You are bleeding more than spotting.
4. Your water breaks.
5. The baby is moving much less than your baseline or not moving at all. If you do kick counts and are able to get the minimum criteria of movements but it still doesn't feel normal for you and your baby's history of movement, call your provider and get evaluated! I have had pregnant people who experienced this exact scenario who were very lucky that they made it in time and their baby was okay. Trust yourself when it comes to this!

REASONS YOU DO NOT NEED TO CALL YOUR PROVIDER
Unless you have a medical reason or your provider has specifically counseled you to do so.

1. You lose your mucus plug.
2. You have spotting in early labor or after intercourse.
3. You are having irregular or mild contractions.
4. You are full term and feel pressure or a fleeting sharp pain in your cervix or pelvis.

ARRIVING AT THE HOSPITAL

When you arrive at the hospital, the baby will be put on the fetal monitor and someone will evaluate you and the baby, which includes a cervical exam to evaluate your progress. Although you may have a pretty good idea that you are transitioning into active labor if the contraction pattern and strength is as described earlier, that is not always the case. Sometimes, depending on the position of the baby, your anatomy, and your natural pain tolerance, you may be much earlier or much later in labor than anticipated. It is common, especially with a first baby, to arrive thinking you must be in active labor only to find that you are 2 centimeters dilated. This can be very frustrating, as you have already gone through so much work in early labor at home, but just know you are definitely not the only one this has happened to.

My first baby was facing my pubic symphysis instead of my sacrum, a position called occiput posterior, and I had a day of intense back labor and only 2 centimeters dilation to show for it. If you are at least 39 weeks, 0 days of pregnancy, and everything looks okay with the baby, you may be given the option of having labor augmented (meaning helped along using the same methods we use during induction), having your cervix reevaluated in two or more hours, or going home and coming back later. Your birth preferences and the amount of pain you are in will help you make the right decision for you. If you arrive and are 4 centimeters or more, admission is typically offered and recommended. Labor usually does not stop at 4 centimeters and you will soon be in active labor. If you arrive at 6 centimeters or more, congratulations! You are in active labor. Labor is more than likely very intense at this point. Some people have the goal of arriving to the hospital in very active labor. Others may wish to arrive as early as possible if they desire pain management for birth or if they are too uncomfortable or unable to bear down or push. Labor can progress rapidly, and the anesthesiologist will be unable to place an epidural if you arrive too late.

PAIN MANAGEMENT

The most common pain management, especially when in active labor, is an epidural. An epidural is a way to deliver anesthesia through a small catheter placed in your lower back. Local numbing medicine is injected first to minimize pain. Most patients feel only pressure when the epidural is placed. To place the epidural catheter, first a needle is inserted in the location where the catheter will be placed. The catheter is threaded into the epidural space, then the needle is removed, leaving only the thin, flexible tubing that is the epidural catheter.

The medication that goes into the catheter is a local anesthetic, or numbing medication, often in combination with a narcotic, or pain medication. Medication is pushed into the catheter by a pump so that you have a constant infusion that numbs your body from the belly button down. You can still feel pressure and may be able to tell when you are having contractions, but the pain should be controlled with the epidural. Because the medication is localized to the epidural space, very little gets to the baby, and there is no evidence of the medication directly causing adverse effects on the baby.

There are many rumors about epidurals, such as that they slow down your labor or wear off so you should wait to get it. Your labor may progress more slowly, not directly due to the epidural, but indirectly: when you cannot feel the pain and move freely, you are less able to intuitively move and shift your body with labor to rotate the baby into the best position to come down into the birth canal. This means that you may need help from the nurses and other support people to change positions or to use birth props if your active stage of labor is moving slowly or your provider decides that the baby is not in the best position. Sometimes, you cannot feel anything when you are fully dilated with an epidural, which can make it hard to push, so you have to wait for the baby to come down more or decrease or stop the flow of medications through the epidural to allow enough sensation to push effectively.

Some women actually progress more quickly in early labor once they get an epidural because they were so tense from pain that their bodies need to relax to allow the cervix to dilate and the baby to come down. You do not have to worry about the epidural running out or wearing off, as additional medication can be added if you begin to feel pain again. Like any procedure, there are risks with an epidural and the anesthesiologist should always discuss all risks (most are extremely rare, such as an infection or a spinal headache) and answer any questions before doing the procedure.

The most common side effect of an epidural is temporary low blood pressure, or hypotension, which may lead to a drop in the baby's heart rate as well. For this reason, IV fluids are given prior to the epidural placement. If you experience a drastic drop in blood pressure after placement, the anesthesiologist may give you medication through your IV to more rapidly increase your blood pressure. Back pain may occur at the site of the epidural for a few days, but there is no evidence of permanent back pain related to epidural placement. Spinal headaches may occur if the spinal needle actually punctures the dura (the covering of the spinal cord), which can lead to leakage of spinal fluid and bad headaches, especially when sitting up. Spinal headaches typically resolve within a few days. If this happens, it is treated with pain medication and occasionally something called a blood patch, in which your own blood is injected into the epidural space to patch the leak and stop the headache.

As an alternative to epidurals, many hospitals also have narcotic sedation available in early labor. This involves a dose of medication through the IV and sometimes in your muscle to help with pain relief. Narcotics are offered only in early labor, as they can sedate the baby if given too close to delivery. Some facilities also offer inhaled gas such as nitrous. This is not as common in the United States as in other countries, but there is momentum growing to start making it more widely available in the United States.

PERSON-CENTERED CARE

Throughout your entire labor course at the hospital, you'll be met with new experiences and considerations, advice from health professionals that may be new or different from what you've heard before, procedures and processes you didn't expect, and perhaps even unanticipated complications. Your comfort, safety, and agency should be honored every step along the way. This is the essence of person-centered care.

Often, there are many options for next steps in your labor course if interventions are recommended. You can discuss the thought process behind your provider's recommendations and let them know if you are comfortable with their plan. Sometimes recommendations are made for safety reasons, sometimes to expedite the labor process, and sometimes based on provider preference or what they have found works best throughout their time in practice. If you do not feel comfortable asking questions and voicing your concerns and preferences, please make sure there is someone in the room with you—whether a partner, friend, family member, or doula—who can be your advocate. Nurses and other support staff in the hospital are also good team members to help you through the process. If you ever feel uncomfortable, make someone aware, because it is always important to understand what is going on and why your provider is recommending certain plans of management.

These pearls of advice from my wonderful colleague and lead midwife at Oula, Saonjie F. Hamilton, certified nurse-midwife, apply not just during labor but throughout your pregnancy and postpartum journey:

> Do not back down. When people say, "I just don't feel right," I take that very seriously. Make sure you are very stern and tell the providers, "I want you to do X, Y, Z." Sometimes people stay with their providers because they feel bad about leaving them. Don't feel intimidated—they are not God—you can ask questions or ask for another provider. Nurses can be excellent advocates—use them! If the doctor says X, Y, Z and leaves the room and you really don't like the plan, talk to the nurse—they are good at connecting with the patient and the provider and offering alternatives. You are not going to mesh with everyone.[2]

WHAT HAPPENS WHEN LABOR STALLS?

When you have planned for a certain labor and birth experience and situations lead to the recommendation for induction, it can be hard to reconcile your birth experience with your expectations. Remember, birth plans are more like birth preferences or wishes. Some interventions are recommended for your safety or for that of your baby.

When recommending an induction, I typically tell patients that this is our first lesson in parenting: we can plan and prepare and envision a certain experience, like when and how we will give birth and exactly how the process will unfold, but our baby teaches us that life involves surprises and changes of plans. You may have to call your boss and tell them that you will not be back to transition projects to a coworker, or call your mother who lives across the country and tell her she needs to fly in sooner, or call the neighbor to let the dog out or to pick up your toddler. I know when I recommend induction it often leads to stress and anxiety due to the loss of control. The unpredictable nature of pregnancy and giving birth can be scary and lead us to want to control every possible aspect, but sometimes we have to lean into the discomfort and uncertainty and trust our bodies and our care team. I am never trying to take away your autonomy or force medical interventions when I recommend an induction. Please remember I am doing it because I truly care about you and your baby and want to make sure both of you have the best possible outcomes.

In the next chapter, we discuss the possible interventions that may be recommended for labor induction. These same methods may also be recommended for augmentation of labor if your labor is not progressing or is progressing very slowly.

THREE

INDUCTION OF LABOR

The following is a very common scenario from my time spent on labor and delivery: I walk into the labor room of a patient who has just arrived for her scheduled induction. We are meeting for the first time. She appears a little nervous but very excited to meet her baby today. She has brought some comfort items from home as well as her partner and other friends and family members. Everyone is ready to go, anticipating that they will be meeting the baby in the next few hours. After I introduce myself and build rapport, I have to reset expectations and explain to them that inductions of labor are long processes. I anticipate that for a first baby, induction will take approximately twenty-four hours from start until birth. I then explain the various methods that may be used for an induction of labor. If the birth person has not heard of these methods, they are often surprised by how complex and variant and arduous the process may be. Sometimes they have solicited the opinions of others in their community or online and have come to the conclusion that many methods of induction are dangerous so they may want to avoid them at all costs.

You can still have a positive birth experience no matter how the labor process starts.

My goal in this chapter is to familiarize you with the common reasons why your provider may recommend an induction of labor as well as the different methods that are commonly used to get you into labor and help labor progress so that you can be ready if an induction is recommended to you. Having your labor induced may be something you hope to avoid, but I promise you can still have a positive birth experience no matter how the labor process starts.

WHAT IS INDUCTION?

An induction of labor is the starting of the labor process before the body does so on its own. Your obstetric provider may recommend your labor to be induced due to a medical reason. You may also be offered the option of an elective induction of labor—that is, you may choose to be induced even if no medical conditions indicate that induction may be needed.

There are several reasons induction of labor may be recommended by your obstetric provider:

* You are getting close to forty-two weeks pregnancy (the recommended cutoff for delivery due to increased stillbirth rate after forty-one weeks of pregnancy).
* Your water broke and you are not in labor.
* Your amniotic fluid level is low.
* You have high blood pressure or preeclampsia.
* You have diabetes.
* Your baby is on the small end of the growth curve (growth restriction).
* Your baby's heart tracing or ultrasound monitoring are concerning enough to recommend delivery but not concerning enough that an urgent C-section is indicated.
* Your placenta is starting to separate from the wall of the uterus (called an abruption), but it is safe for you to try for a vaginal birth.
* Countless other maternal or fetal indications.

ELECTIVE INDUCTIONS

For many birthing people, avoiding induction of labor is a top priority. More physiologic techniques, such as exercise, intercourse, and acupuncture have all been tried, as well as the consumption of everything from an abundance of dates to very spicy foods or other edible substances such as primrose oil and castor oil. There is even a salad made in Los Angeles that is touted to send those who consume it into labor.[1] It is hard to determine the actual efficacy of these methods since there are many other confounding factors, and your body simply may have been ready to go into labor (after all, you should never try to start labor prior to thirty-nine weeks without a medical indication).

Whether or not you have attempted every possible means to avoid an induction of labor, choosing to be induced—regardless of whether it's medically recommended by your doctor—actually has been shown to decrease the risks of many of the common complications that you may have thought were associated with an induction.

In 2018, a large, multi-institutional study called the ARRIVE trial looked at the birth outcomes of women induced electively at thirty-nine weeks versus waiting for spontaneous labor up to forty-one weeks of pregnancy. C-section rates were significantly lower among women who had a low Bishop score (indicating an unripe cervix—more on this later) who were randomized to have an elective induction of labor at thirty-nine weeks than women who were randomized to the expectant management group (waiting up to forty-one weeks for spontaneous labor).[2] There were also significantly lower rates of gestational hypertension, preeclampsia, neonatal respiratory support, and NICU stays among the induction group. We know that the placenta ages as you progress into late-term pregnancy, which is why the risk of stillbirth and severe fetal morbidity are high enough by forty-two weeks to recommend delivery prior to that point. But even before then, if the placenta is not working as well, babies are less likely to tolerate labor, leading to a C-section. They are also more likely to have meconium, or the first stool, in the amniotic fluid, which can lead to more NICU stays for respiratory support and monitoring due to complications of meconium getting into their lungs. We also know that the further you get into pregnancy, the greater the chances of high blood pressure and preeclampsia developing, so your chance of developing one of these pregnancy complications increases the longer you remain pregnant past thirty-nine weeks.

Due to these findings, the American College of Obstetricians and Gynecologists now states that it is reasonable for obstetricians and health-care facilities to offer elective induction of labor to low-risk, first-time birthing people at thirty-nine weeks gestation. This study has caused a big shift among institutions and providers that have the resources to allow for elective inductions of labor at thirty-nine weeks, which now offer this as a routine option for any patient who desires an elective induction of labor.

I spoke to one of my amazing colleagues, Saonjie Hamilton, certified nurse-midwife, a lead midwife at Oula, a midwife-led collaborative care practice in New York. Saonjie has been practicing obstetrics for fifteen years. Having had the privilege of working beside her on labor and delivery, I admire her and how she cares for our patients tremendously. Because midwives are experts in physiological birth (or natural birth), I asked Saonjie how she approaches the topic of a medically indicated induction of labor with our patients. Here's what she said:

> Sometimes things don't go as planned. If nothing else, the [COVID-19] pandemic has taught us that. I ask [my patient], what is your ultimate end goal? Is it to avoid an induction? Is it to have a vaginal birth? Is it to have a safe delivery? A good baby? A good mommy? [If they are a Black or Brown person] I acknowledge that [for many valid reasons], Black and Brown people do not trust the medical industrial complex, but there's a reason you came to us; you trust us and you trust that we have your best interest at heart. The reality is that Black patients have a higher morbidity and mortality, and if we can avoid that, we are going to do that.[3]

PREPARING FOR YOUR INDUCTION OF LABOR

I have had many shifts on labor and delivery when patients who are admitted for induction of labor are not prepared for the process or the amount of time to expect from the start of an induction of labor until the birth. They often arrive with their partners and multiple friends and family members, anticipating that the baby will arrive within a few hours. Unless you have had a few babies and your cervix is already very ripe when you arrive, this is extremely unlikely to be the case.

Inductions of labor can take a long time. Once the induction process starts, it is reasonable to anticipate approximately twenty-four hours until delivery for your first baby. Consider yourself lucky if the process moves along more quickly than this; do not consider it a failure if it takes longer. A failed induction means that you have been induced for twenty-four hours and are not yet in active labor or that you have been on Pitocin and had your water broken for twelve to eighteen hours and are not yet in active labor. Active labor starts at 6 centimeters of dilation. This means that some women are only 6 centimeters dilated at the twenty-four-hour mark after being induced. From this point, average dilation in the active stage is 1 to 2 centimeters per hour followed by, on average, two hours of pushing for a first baby. None of these time frames are the outer limits; if you have a bigger baby or smaller pelvis, if you are obese, or if the baby is not in the best position to come down the birth canal, active labor and pushing may take even longer. I say all of this to let you know that you should come prepared to be at the hospital for a while. Eat a good meal and take a nice shower before you come; depending on your hospital protocol, you may not be allowed to eat regular food from the time you arrive until you deliver. Bring plenty of entertainment: books, music, shows or movies you have been too busy to watch, whatever helps you happily pass the time. You are in it for the long haul, so please do not be frustrated or disappointed when things do not happen quickly.

When you are being induced, there are a few other things you should expect:

- You will need an IV and will often be on IV fluids.
- You will need to stay on the fetal monitor because your providers must be able to see the baby's heartbeat and your contraction pattern when you are being induced.
- Your mobility will be decreased compared to laboring at home or even in the hospital when you have spontaneous labor.

As Saonjie tells her patients, "When you are coming in for an induction, you need to understand that with an induction of labor they can't avoid interventions—that's what an induction is. I am fully transparent. Make sure your mind is ready for it."

INDUCTION OF LABOR METHODS

How you are induced will depend on your cervical exam. The changes to your cervix—how soft, thin, and open it is—your cervix's position in the vagina, and how low the baby is (station) all add up to a measurement called the Bishop score. The Bishop score was defined and published by Dr. E. H. Bishop in 1964 in his article titled "Pelvic Scoring for Elective Induction." This scoring system is still routinely used today. A Bishop score is typically calculated based on your vaginal exam when you arrive for an induction of labor. The higher your Bishop score, the more "ripe" or favorable your cervix is, and typically the easier it will be to get labor started. A score of eight or more is considered favorable, and often induction will be started with oxytocin or by amniotomy (artificial rupture of membranes). A score of six or lower is considered unfavorable, and induction is typically started with a ripening agent, such as a cervical ripening balloon or prostaglandins. Descriptions of all methods of induction and what to anticipate with each follow. You can go to Perinatalology.com to see the Bishop score calculator and even use it to calculate your own score when your provider examines your cervix.[4]

The following methods of getting you into labor and helping your labor progress may be recommended to you throughout your induction course. The more you familiarize yourself with them now, the less scary and confusing it may be when you are presented with one or many options in the hospital.

Prostaglandins

If your cervix is not ripe, induction is typically started with prostaglandins such as Cervidil (dinoprostone) or Cytotec (misoprostol), both of which may be placed vaginally. Sometimes Cytotec is placed in your cheek and then swallowed. Prostaglandins mimic the natural inflammatory factors that are released when your body goes into labor and help ripen the cervix to get labor started. These medications may be used alone or in combination with a cervical ripening balloon. Cytotec is used off-label when it is used to induce labor. This means that the Food and Drug Administration (FDA) has not approved it specifically for inducing labor. It has been extensively studied, however, and is one of the most common medications used for labor induction. There are many medications in use that may be used for non-FDA-approved reasons, but this does not mean that they are unsafe. Cervidil, a prostaglandin that is FDA approved for cervical ripening, is much more expensive than misoprostol, so many hospitals have only misoprostol available.

Cervical Ripening Balloon

A cervical ripening balloon is a catheter with two empty balloons on one end. The catheter is threaded through your cervix and into the lower portion of the uterus, and the two balloons are filled, one above the cervix and one below, to put pressure on either side of the cervix, which mechanically compresses and stretches your cervix. If your hospital does not have the trademarked Cook Cervical Ripening Balloon, it may use a foley catheter, which is similar and used regularly in the bladder to drain urine. For induction, it is used in a similar way to the Cook balloon. The difference is that the foley catheter has only one balloon, which is inflated inside the cervix instead of two that put pressure on the cervix from both sides. Both may be inserted with the aid of a speculum or your provider may insert it using their hands (as they would when doing a cervical exam). If you're curious about how a Cook Cervical Ripening Balloon or a foley catheter works for induction of labor, there are good educational videos available on YouTube.

If the process of having a cervical ripening balloon placed sounds uncomfortable, that's because it is. This method causes a lot of cramping and pressure. Many people request pain management either before or during the procedure. Based on conversations with my patients, the pain tends to be the worst during placement and the first thirty minutes after placement, then they tend to adjust to the pressure and cramping. This doesn't mean that they forget the balloon is there—you will feel it if you don't have anesthesia until it comes out.

Typically, the balloon is checked every few hours until your cervix has dilated to approximately 5 centimeters and the balloon falls out. This does not, however, mean that you will progress rapidly into active labor. Often, when the balloon falls out, you are still not having strong regular contractions, your cervix has not thinned out, and the baby has not come down. This means that your cervix has been stretched open, but your body has not caught up yet with the physiologic progression to active labor. The time elapsed between a 5-centimeter cervical ripening balloon cervix and a 6-centimeter active labor cervix may be lengthy.

Pitocin

Pitocin, the IV medication that mimics your natural oxytocin, is a medication that may be recommended after the prostaglandins have dilated your cervix or even initially in conjunction with a cervical ripening balloon. Pitocin has developed a bad reputation over the years, because it makes contractions very strong. If used too aggressively, contractions may become too frequent or too strong, which may lead to distress to the baby or even a rupture of the uterus. Due to these risks, hospitals have protocols for how to safely start and increase or decrease Pitocin based on the baby's heart rate pattern and the contraction pattern. If used safely, Pitocin can help you progress in labor when natural contractions are not strong or frequent enough.

Rupture of Membranes (aka "Breaking Your Water")

During the induction process, your provider may recommend breaking your water for you instead of waiting for it to break spontaneously, a process called artificial rupture of membranes. It may be recommended at any point in the labor course; practice and preferences between providers and hospitals vary considerably. I always tell my patients that unless labor has stalled, we do not have to break the water. Unless necessary as a last resort for getting a patient into labor, I never recommend breaking the water until the baby's head is well applied to the cervix. If the baby's head is too high, there is risk of what is called cord prolapse: the baby's umbilical cord can slip below the head with the gush of fluid when the water is broken. When the head comes down, it presses on the umbilical cord, and the baby cannot get oxygen. This is cause for an emergency cesarean section. The benefits of breaking the water are that it can decrease the time until delivery and help to progress stalled labor. The contractions become much stronger and more painful once your water is broken. In addition to cord prolapse, there are other risks: once the cushion of fluid is gone, the umbilical cord can be compressed more easily with contractions, which can lead to non-reassuring fetal heart tracing (the baby not tolerating contractions), as well as increased risk of infection once the barrier between vaginal bacteria and the uterus is gone (especially if you have multiple cervical exams after the water is broken).

If your water breaks naturally at home, there is less risk of cord prolapse. Often, (1) you haven't even started labor and your cervix is minimally dilated, so the umbilical cord has less chance of slipping through the cervix, or (2) you are in active labor spontaneously and typically when that happens your baby's head has already dropped low enough to act as a cork stop, blocking the cord from slipping below the baby's head. That said, always call your provider immediately if your water breaks at home to make a plan for coming to the hospital.

Membrane Sweep (aka Stripping the Membranes)

A method of induction that may be done in the doctor's office is called membrane stripping or sweeping the membranes. This separates the amniotic membranes from the cervix, which causes your body's natural prostaglandins to be released. When your body is ready to go into labor, it initiates the process. If your body is not ready, you may have cramping, contractions, and spotting that stops and does not progress to labor. If your cervix is not dilated, this cannot be done, because your provider must be able to get a finger inside of the cervix to separate the cervix from the bag of water.

Nipple Stimulation

Nipple stimulation may also be recommended as a more natural means of induction, as this releases oxytocin, which can start contractions.

This may be done manually or with a breast pump. This is not an active method of induction of labor used in the hospital, and I discourage my patients from employing this at home, because it can cause frequent contractions, and we cannot monitor the baby from home to ensure the baby is tolerating the contractions.

INDUCTIONS SAVE LIVES

An induction of labor can save your and your baby's life in certain scenarios. Early in my training, I was involved in the care of a young woman who developed preeclampsia at thirty-seven weeks of pregnancy. This was prior to the change in recommendations from induction between thirty-seven and thirty-nine weeks for preeclampsia without severe features (meaning she had only mildly elevated blood pressures and protein in her urine, without other symptoms or lab abnormalities) to the new standard to induce everyone with preeclampsia without severe features at thirty-seven weeks of pregnancy. It was also prior to the ARRIVE trial. Her cervical exam was unfavorable, meaning her cervix had not yet ripened, which we thought at the time meant that it would be harder to get labor started and she would have a higher risk of cesarean section. The plan was made to monitor her and her baby closely over the next two weeks, giving her body more time to prepare for labor, and then to induce labor at thirty-nine weeks if she did not develop preeclampsia with severe features prior.

Tragically, at thirty-eight weeks of pregnancy, she suddenly developed severe high blood pressure and had a placental abruption, in which the placenta separates from the wall of the uterus, and her baby died. She lost a lot of blood and could have died as well if she did not come immediately to the hospital when she felt that something was wrong. With her subsequent pregnancy, her blood pressure started to rise again around thirty-seven weeks. This time, there were no thoughts about waiting. She came in for an induction of labor, and after an uncomplicated labor, she gave birth to a beautiful, healthy baby.

I will never forget this patient or either of her babies. I did the ultrasound when she came in after the abruption, and I had to tell her the baby had died. I was present when she birthed her stillborn baby. I also followed her closely during her second pregnancy and was present when she birthed her beautiful, healthy, crying baby. Her story has shaped many aspects of the way I view obstetrics and connect with my patients. It also changed the way I viewed inductions. Many birthing people are wary of inductions, but when looking at the big picture, sometimes an induction can mean the difference between life and death. I hope I never have to hand another parent a stillborn baby when an induction could have meant handing them a live baby.

Once you have gone into labor either spontaneously or with an induction, the next step is the second stage of labor: giving birth! I'm sure you have dreamed of your baby's birth for a long time, and now that it's finally here, let's get into the details of what that may look and feel like. In the next chapter, we explore the second stage of labor and delve into the incredible experience of birthing your baby.

FOUR

VAGINAL BIRTH

We have thought about the common narratives of how labor should start and progress, but what about the birth itself? If you go on social media, what is the image of an ideal birth that you see? What did you envision when making your birth plan? Have you allowed for the possibility that your birth story may not go according to your expectations? What makes a birth a "good birth"? How can you feel like you had a good birth even if it doesn't match your ideal birth experience? Good birth isn't how it *looks*—it's how you feel about it. Knowing what to realistically expect during the second stage of labor will help you feel better about the things that may otherwise have been surprising and upsetting.

The time it takes from full dilation to meeting your baby can vary significantly. I have seen birth parents become very frustrated or disillusioned because, despite being told that they are "so close" and "doing great," they have been pushing for hours and it seems like nothing is happening. I have also had many birth parents tell me they "can't do it," or they want me to just "take the baby out" because they feel they are not strong enough or they can't wrap their mind around how their baby will come out of their vagina. These moments test your physical strength, but they also test your emotional and mental capacity to trust in yourself, your body, and the awe-inspiring act of giving birth.

One of the most fulfilling and amazing aspects of my profession is that I get to witness, over and over again, the transformation in someone who thinks they can't do it but then successfully pushes their baby out and meets their baby for the first time. This is such an empowering experience. I have even seen the process of giving birth help transform women who were sexually abused in the past and had disassociated with their bodies in many ways to see themselves, their bodies, their personal strength, and their autonomy in a totally new way after taking back ownership of their bodies and discovering their own innate power and the miraculous way they are capable of bringing a new life into the world. To witness this transition—this transformation—and see the look of awe on someone's face when they behold their own power and what they have brought forth into the world is beyond words. It makes me feel so lucky and honored to bear witness to this process every single time.

> *To witness this transition— this transformation—and see the look of awe on someone's face when they behold their own power and what they have brought forth into the world is beyond words.*

STAGE 2: PUSHING

In chapter 2, we discussed stage 1 of labor, both the latent (up to 5 centimeters dilated) and active (6–10 centimeters dilated) stages. Once fully dilated, you enter stage 2 of labor. It may be recommended to start pushing right away, or your provider may recommend something called "laboring down," which means passively allowing the baby to move further down the birth canal on their own. This is much harder to do without anesthesia. With an epidural—especially if you are very numb and/or the baby is still not very low in the pelvis—laboring down may be recommended to decrease the overall time spent pushing to avoid wearing yourself out. Studies have shown that laboring down does not decrease cesarean sections, so the decision about whether to labor down is often a discussion between patient and provider about what may be best for their particular situation.

Often, if a birthing person wants to try some practice pushes, I guide them and see how well they are able to push for a few contractions. If it seems that they are too numb and unable to push effectively, I have them relax and rest and recheck them in an hour to allow the epidural to wear off some and the baby to move lower so that they are able to push more effectively. If the baby's heart rate is concerning at all, if the birth person has developed an infection in the uterus, or if they show other complications such as bleeding or anything else that precludes waiting to start pushing, the provider may recommend turning down the epidural so that pushing can be effective sooner.

Pushing is not like in the movies. Unless you have had a baby (or a few) prior, it is extremely rare to start pushing and give birth within a few pushes. It is common to become discouraged when it seems like you aren't progressing; however, most of the time, it takes at least a few hours to get to the point of crowning, especially with a first birth. The early work involves relaxation of the pelvic floor and molding of the baby's head. The relaxation of the pelvic floor occurs as the baby puts pressure on the muscles and ligaments of your pelvic floor and is enhanced with pushing. Molding is how babies get what is called a "cone head" and is also the reason why they have soft spots in their head at birth; the bones need to be able to mold and overlap to help the baby squeeze through the pelvic bones.

Pushing will be very different depending on whether you have pain control or not, and if you do, what type of pain control you are receiving. If you are giving birth without any pain medication, you will feel the urge and the intensity of the contractions, which aid in knowing when to push and where to focus your pushing efforts. You may also intuitively move into positions that feel better to you and help the baby rotate in your pelvis. This is why giving birth without pain medication often involves less time pushing than with pain medication. If you are receiving an epidural or another form of pain management, it can be harder to feel where to push and even to know when your contractions are occurring. The majority of people giving birth in the hospital do utilize some form of analgesic, epidurals being the most common. Do not get discouraged if you know you will want an epidural or if you decide in labor to get an epidural or alternative pain management. Sometimes the medication needs to be decreased or turned off completely to regain enough sensation to push effectively; however, sometimes the birth person is able to push in the right place to make progress during the second stage of labor without much sensation of what they are doing.

Pushing may seem very intuitive, but it involves a lot of coordination between relaxing the pelvic floor and engaging the abdominal core. It often takes some time to get the hang of it, especially if you have an epidural and cannot feel the sensation to get proper feedback and know whether you are engaging your core muscles. Having a good coach—either your nurse, doula, or provider—to provide that feedback at first is important and helps you to know when you are pushing effectively. Pelvic floor physical therapy can be beneficial prior to giving birth, so that you understand the muscles to engage and the muscles to relax when pushing before going to labor and delivery.

When you are pushing, you may feel like nothing is happening. This is because early pushing requires the pelvic floor to stretch and the baby's head to rotate and mold to fit under the pubic bone. The baby often gently rocks back and forth with pushes and is making a slow descent, which can be frustrating—it may be an hour or so before you can really tell that the baby has moved lower in the birth canal. Once the baby fits under the pubic bone, the pressure and pain can become much more intense as the labia separate and the opening to the vagina stretches. At this point, birth parents often feel a burning sensation due to the stretching and may be afraid to push, because it feels impossible that their vagina will survive the baby coming through the opening. At this point, you just have to trust that your body can do this and that your vagina and perineum will not explode. You have to push through the intense pain; if you hold back your pushing effort, it only protracts the second stage and you will feel the intense pressure and burning pain for even longer.

When your baby crowns, or extends their head to exit through the opening of the vagina, your provider may give you some directions to slow or pause the pushing at certain times. This is to help the opening of the vagina to stretch more slowly and decrease tearing. However, if the baby shows signs of stress, which sometimes happens during pushing, you may be encouraged to push with all of your strength and birth your baby as quickly as possible. Just listen to their advice and if you have any questions, please ask.

As mentioned earlier, pushing takes an average of two hours with a first baby but can be faster or slower. There is no definitive upper limit of pushing as long as progress is made (i.e., the baby is continuing to descend in the birth canal). Usually, though, the birth parent is fatigued by the three to four hour mark, or the baby may begin to show signs of stress, and then it is recommended to expedite delivery with an operative delivery or a cesarean section, depending on how low the baby is in the birth canal. Additionally, a prolonged second stage increases the risk of hemorrhage, or excessive bleeding, so this must be taken into account if you have a long second stage. Figure 4.1 provides a great visual of fetal station, or how low the baby is in your pelvis, so that you can better understand what your provider is referring to.

If this is not your first baby, you may be pleasantly surprised, because the time for both the first and the second stages of labor tend to progress much more rapidly with subsequent babies. I have cared for many birth people who had unpleasant experiences and even trauma with their first birth due to a long second stage, operative delivery, and/or a bad perineal tear, and they were able to avoid all of this with the second birth. Once the birth canal has been navigated by one baby,

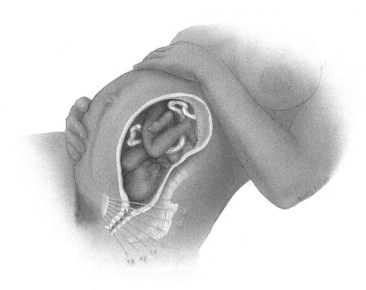

Figure 4.1. Birth Stations. *Biotic Artlab, 2024*

it stretches to accommodate the next baby much more easily, so all of the time spent relaxing the pelvic floor muscles is not needed again.

Once the baby's head has delivered, the rest of the body typically delivers easily.

POSSIBLE COMPLICATIONS DURING LABOR

Becoming fully dilated does not guarantee a spontaneous vaginal birth. If you have had a vaginal birth prior, your chances of having a spontaneous vaginal birth at this point are pretty good; however, there are still some situations that, no matter your prior births, may lead your care team to recommend an operative vaginal birth or a cesarean birth.

Signs of Distress

Let's go back to the basics a bit to understand what your provider is thinking when you are in the second stage of labor. We are always looking at your baby's heart rate, your status (your energy, pushing effort, and vital signs, for example), and how you are progressing (how the baby is coming down the birth canal) when you are pushing. If your baby's heart rate tracing shows concerning signs in labor or for fetal distress (referred to as a "non-reassuring fetal heart tracing"), this may limit the time of the second stage. Every time you contract, blood flow to the uterus—and therefore the delivery of oxygenated blood through the placenta to your baby—is limited. Pushing increases the stress on your baby, decreasing the flow of oxygenated blood through the placenta even further.

Every baby's threshold for stress is different and influenced by many factors, most importantly how well your placenta is functioning, as well as factors such as whether the umbilical cord is being compressed during contractions. This means that if your baby starts to show signs of distress when you are pushing, we may recommend changing your position, giving you oxygen or IV fluids, stopping Pitocin, giving you medication to stop contractions for a short period of time, or laboring down (take a break from pushing) or pushing with every other contraction. The recommendations depend on what appears to be the underlying cause of the tracing abnormalities. If the baby's heart rate still does not recover or worsens, your provider will make an assessment based on the baby's overall tracing, as well as on the station and position of your baby (how low the baby is in your pelvis and which way they are facing), the size of your baby, and whether or not you have diabetes (the last two factors being red flags for shoulder dystocia), while taking into account whether you have had vaginal births before.

Prior vaginal births—especially if the baby is already descending quickly—may mean that your team thinks that you can deliver very quickly without any assistance and without risk of prolonged fetal distress. They will then let you know if an operative delivery is an option or whether a C-section is recommended. Certain factors may make it too risky for the baby to even try an operative delivery with the assistance of vacuum or forceps. Even if that is an option, whether a vacuum-assisted delivery and/or forceps is the best option and is available will influence the way you are counseled. Even if an operative vaginal delivery is an option and is available, parents sometimes prefer to proceed with a cesarean birth rather than attempting an operative vaginal delivery.

The course of action when a baby is in distress has to be decided quickly; however, you should always feel that you have received adequate counseling and understand the risks, benefits, and alternatives of your options before proceeding. I discussed the risks of C-section earlier and operative deliveries in chapter 1, and I talk more about C-sections in chapter 5. It is always best to receive and understand this information at a time when you can process it and ask questions of your provider in a more relaxed setting as opposed to having the often stressful conversations and decisions to make while you are in labor.

Maternal Complications

Besides fetal indications for expediting delivery, there also may be maternal indications. The birthing person may have underlying cardiac or pulmonary conditions, in which case they may not have the stamina to spend a lot of time pushing. Occasionally, due to the maternal risks of labor and pushing, a passive vaginal birth (no pushing, often assisted via forceps) or a scheduled cesarean section is recommended.

The whole labor process, especially the second stage, is phys-iologically intense, like running a marathon. And just as baby may become distressed, moms with certain conditions may also become distressed. Besides preexisting medical conditions, birthing people may also develop severe range blood pressures and other symptoms of preeclampsia that may indicate induction of labor; however, if they worsen during labor and expedited delivery is recommended, this can occur at any point during labor or pushing and may lead to the recom-mendation for an operative delivery or cesarean section. If you have severe range blood pressures or other symptoms of preeclampsia, you will be closely monitored in labor and counseled if delivery needs to be expedited to avoid serious maternal and fetal complications.

Another situation that may occur is an abruption, in which the placenta starts to separate from the wall of the uterus. This can happen prior to labor and be an indication for delivery or it may happen at any point during the labor process. Delivery recommendations in this instance are made based on both maternal and fetal status. If there is evidence of fetal distress or maternal bleeding that puts the birth parent at risk of hemorrhage, your doctor will recommend a C-section or operative birth, depending on the circumstances.

Other indications for an operative delivery or C-section may be when birth parent and baby are both stable, but the birthing person has been pushing for a prolonged period and the baby either is not descending or is descending slowly. Other times, the birthing person may be exhausted and request an expedited delivery via one of these means. As I said before, labor and pushing are physically taxing. When undergoing one of the most strenuous activities of your life while sleep deprived and not eating, many people become too tired to keep pushing after a few hours.

There is no definitive cutoff for how long someone can be fully dilated or can push before they must give birth. However, the longer someone is pushing, the higher the risk for hemorrhage after delivery, and the longer someone is in labor with their water broken, the higher the risk of developing an infection (chorioamnionitis). Therefore, if no or minimal progress is made after one or two hours, the provider may recommend intervention earlier than if slow but steady progress is being made over three to four hours.

Shoulder Dystocia

In the rare case of a shoulder dystocia, in which the baby's shoulders and abdomen are wider than the head, your provider may have to do some extra maneuvers to help deliver your baby. Again, they should let you know what is going on. Most shoulder dystocia maneuvers take a minute or less. Occasionally, some may take longer, require more maneuvers, and extra people may be brought into the room to assist, including a pediatrician. It can be scary because things move quickly when a shoulder dystocia is diagnosed and multiple people are doing a lot of things at the same time; however, the goal is to get your baby delivered as soon as possible, because every minute the baby is not born after the head is delivered means another minute your baby is not getting oxygen. Most of the time, these maneuvers involve changing your position to make more space for the baby, applying pressure above your pubic bone to release the baby's shoulder, and occasionally having a provider dislodge the shoulder that is stuck with their hands inside of your vagina. Rarely an episiotomy will be recommended to assist with these maneuvers. All of this happens very quickly, and if you do not have an epidural, it can be painful—even with an epidural, you may feel more pressure and pain if the epidural has worn off significantly while pushing. Your team's goal is to deliver your baby safely; once your baby is safe and being evaluated by the pediatricians, they will discuss exactly what happened and answer all questions.

Infection

Intraamniotic infection (IAI) is the most common infection encountered during labor. This is an infection inside the uterus and may involve the amniotic sac, amniotic fluid, placenta, umbilical cord, or the baby itself. It is most likely to occur with a long labor, especially when the amniotic sac has been ruptured for a prolonged time period (called prolonged rupture of the membranes). The first sign of this infection is usually a fever and is often accompanied by a high heart rate in the baby and/or birthing person. When an IAI is diagnosed, IV fluids, antibiotics, and Tylenol are given to treat the infection and lower baby's heart rate to a normal range. Infection itself is not a reason to move toward a cesarean birth; however, the infection can make it more difficult to achieve a vaginal birth, and with a prolonged infection, there is a higher risk of the infection spreading to the baby. Infection can make the uterus contract less efficiently, making it hard to achieve adequate contractions to make cervical change and become fully dilated. Also, if the baby's heart rate stays very elevated for a prolonged time, it can stress the baby, leading to non-reassuring fetal heart rate, which may be an indication to expedite delivery via cesarean birth.

When you have an IAI, you will have to ask your care team about the hospital's protocol for treating the baby after birth. Hospitals have different protocols in place to help prevent neonatal sepsis, which may include observation and antibiotics in the NICU for the baby. Hospitals often use a sepsis score to determine your baby's risk for sepsis, which takes into account factors such as the highest temperature you had in labor, how long your membranes were ruptured prior to delivery, and if your group B strep was positive. I mention this because it is important to understand that even if your baby comes out looking great and has a normal temperature, they still may be admitted to the NICU for antibiotics and close monitoring. Babies have very weak immune systems and cannot easily fight infections, so those with a high risk for infection may be admitted to the NICU preventatively, even if they are not yet showing any signs of infection.

Meconium

This is the first poop of the newborn baby. Although most babies pass their first stool after being born (sometimes even while being squeezed out of the vagina!), some babies pass meconium while still inside the uterus. This is commonly related to a few different situations.

1. You are past your due date. The further you get past your due date (also called "post-dates"), the greater the chance that the baby will pass their first stool while still inside the uterus.
2. The baby was stressed while inside the uterus and passed stool. This can happen when there were signs of a non-reassuring fetal tracing or concern for fetal distress before delivery. This does not, however, mean that your baby will have abnormal cord blood gas or signs or symptoms of permanent damage from this stress.

Often, it is known before delivery that the baby has pooped inside the uterus. This is because once your water is broken, the fluid that comes out through your vagina will be mixed with the meconium. When you are evaluated after spontaneously breaking your water or a provider artificially breaks your water, they will note if the fluid is clear or if there is meconium. If meconium is present, they may also note if it is thin, moderate, or thick. The thicker the meconium, the more concern there is that the baby will get meconium into their lungs when they take their first breaths. Sometimes we do not detect meconium until delivery, when we can see it on the baby or in the fluid that comes out after birth. If the baby's head is already engaged in your pelvis when they poop, the meconium may not leak out of the vagina, so your provider or nurse may note meconium on the baby's skin. If there is any amount of meconium, your care team will let you and the NICU team know. They are typically called to do immediate suctioning and additional resuscitation if it appears that the baby did get some meconium into their lungs. Sometimes the baby can go immediately skin-to-skin, depending on how your baby looks when born and the hospital's protocols; however, often the baby has to be taken to the warmer in your delivery room for closer evaluation, suctioning, and possibly further resuscitation. If your care team tells you that meconium is present, ask them about the facility's typical protocol so that you are prepared if the baby is taken immediately to the warmer for evaluation.

The main thing to know about meconium is that it does not mean that there is anything wrong with your baby. If meconium combined with concerning fetal heart tracing was noted prior to delivery, that could indicate that the baby was probably under some level of distress and pooped inside as a result—but again, that does *not* mean that your baby is still distressed after birth or will suffer any long-term consequences from the stress inside the uterus. No matter the reason for meconium, it is important that the care team works as quickly as possible to make sure your baby's mouth and nose are clear of meconium so that it does not get into your baby's lungs. If it is suspected that meconium is in the lungs, the baby will be taken to the NICU for observation and sometimes given supplemental oxygen if they are showing signs of difficulty breathing and antibiotics to prevent an infection from developing in their lungs. Again, babies have very weak immune systems and do not have a lot of respiratory reserve (they get tired very easily if they are laboring to breathe), so extra caution is always taken. This separation and concern is always difficult for new birth parents. Just know your baby is getting the attention and support they need to safely go home with you when discharged from the NICU.

Perineal Tears

During the second stage of labor, you may have tearing on the vulva, in the vagina, or outside the vagina on the perineum. Perineal tears, which are tears between the opening to the vagina toward (or into) the rectum, are the most common type of tears. However, you may also have tearing inside the vagina and more rarely on the labia, cervix, or near your urethra (through which you pee) or clitoris. All of this depends on the size, position, and manner at which your baby exits your pelvis as well as your pelvic anatomy. I discuss repair and recovery after tearing in a later chapter. Please see figure 4.2 for the four different categories of perineal tears.

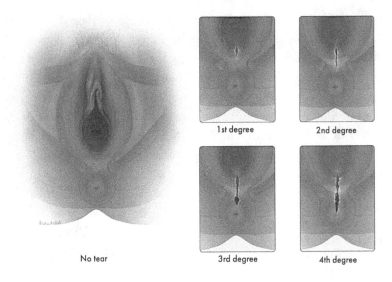

Figure 4.2. Perineal Tears. *Biotic Artlab, 2024*

WHAT WOULD YOU DO?

Just as with medicine more generally, some recommendations are evidence based and standardized across the medical practice, whereas others must be individualized for the patient, taking into account the health needs and preferences of that particular birthing person. The lack of standardization and definitive criteria may be freeing and encouraging to some people, whereas others become distressed and want a definitive recommendation or plan from their provider. I have often had patients ask me, "What would you do if you were in my situation?"

I tell them that I have my own lived experience and made decisions based on my body and my babies. I can tell you what I think I would do in your situation, but (1) you never know the right decision for another person unless you are in their shoes, and (2) that may not be the best decision for someone else, even if it would be the best decision for me. You may feel forced to make a decision that you are not certain about. It's possible that, after the fact and knowing the outcome, we might look back and feel that we have made the wrong decision. So I always tell people that when they have multiple options with which their provider feels comfortable—meaning none is recommended over the others—then they have to decide what feels right for them. Retrospectively you may learn more information that might have changed your decision, but try your best not to make yourself feel bad after the fact. Life is full of uncertainties. Often, being pregnant and giving birth are the first times we are faced directly with the feeling of loss of control and not being 100 percent sure about our decisions, which can be very scary. But the truth is, we are never really in control of outcomes. All we can do is the best we can with the information we have at the time (and be sure that your care team answers all of your questions to your satisfaction prior to making your decision), and then we use our logical reasoning plus our gut instincts to make that choice. Easier said than done, but trust me, when you have kids at home, your whole life becomes a practice of doing the best you can with the information you have at the time.

When you have kids at home, your whole life becomes a practice of doing the best you can with the information you have at the time.

IMMEDIATELY AFTER BIRTH

If your baby or your delivery involves any complications that require the pediatricians to be at the birth, then they will be called when you are close to delivering. Depending on the situation, there may be one person or multiple people from the NICU at the birth, as well as the baby nurse, a nurse from labor and delivery who is present at all births, since your primary nurse is caring for you. If your baby does not require immediate evaluation by the pediatricians or the baby nurse, then the baby should be placed skin-to-skin directly on you (unless, of course, you request that the baby be taken to the warmer). Delayed cord clamping is also routine at this point in time due to its known benefits, though practices may vary. Some places delay for one minute, as a majority of the benefits have been received at this point, and other places delay until the cord has stopped pulsating. At this point, the cord is clamped and cut by one of your support people or your provider. If your baby comes out and requires immediate evaluation by the pediatric team or if the cord is tight around the baby's neck, delayed cord clamping may not be possible.

Birthing your baby is a time of extreme vulnerability. Often people describe a sense of feeling out of control and simply allowing their animalistic nature take over. Some people embrace this; others hate the feeling of being out of control. Birth can feel like a beautiful, empowering experience—or a brutal, horrific experience. You may feel all of these emotions at the same time, as well as other complex and nuanced emotions. Everything you feel during your birth and the aftermath when you process it is completely valid, not just the nice, socially acceptable feelings.

No matter what your friends and family members have told you, you cannot appreciate the depths and range of the emotions you will feel once you birth your baby and witness the power of the female body and mind—the accomplishment of something that hours or minutes before may have seemed completely impossible. To watch someone undergo that transformation in real time—seeing the look on their face and feeling the shift in energy in the room once they have accomplished one of the hardest things they will ever do in life—is so incredibly awe inspiring. Every time I bear witness to a birth, I am reminded of why I fell in love with obstetrics in the first place.

FIVE

CESAREAN BIRTH

I recently cared for a patient who had gone for her thirty-nine week appointment with one of the midwives at my practice and was told her blood pressure was high. The midwife recommended that she come to labor and delivery for an induction of labor. The patient had hoped for spontaneous labor, but after all of her questions were answered, she accepted this change to her plan and came in for an induction. Once she got into labor, she rapidly progressed and reached 6 centimeters dilation very quickly. At this point, I had just met the patient, because the midwife was managing her induction. I was there for backup in case an obstetrician was needed.

Suddenly, her baby's heart rate dropped significantly. For approximately six minutes, the team worked furiously using every possible intervention to try to resuscitate the baby and return the baby's heart rate to the baseline. I explained to her that I recommended going to the operating room and then reassessing the baby's heart rate. If the heart rate was normal by the time we got into the operating room (OR), we could monitor her there for a short period and then return to the labor room. If the baby's heart rate was still low, however, then the safest thing to do for her baby would be to have a cesarean birth.

The birth patient calmly agreed to the plan and we rushed to the OR. The baby's heart rate remained low, and the decision was made to proceed with the cesarean birth. We conducted the emergency operation swiftly, because we did not want to risk stressing the baby. The birth patient's partner and midwife stayed next to her throughout the surgery, and she was able to see the baby immediately after birth. She and her baby both did very well. Afterward, when I was speaking to her in the recovery area, she was calm and accepting of the outcome and grateful that they were both okay. I saw her again the next morning and asked how she felt about the cesarean birth and if she had any questions. She said that she had accepted during her pregnancy that certain things were out of her control, and she felt that she and her baby were well cared for and had a good outcome. She did not have any signs of stress or trauma from the experience.

It wasn't the birth she wanted, but it was the birth she *needed*.

Many of my patients' births have gone off course from their plans, but if they were prepared for and accepting of the fact that many elements of birth are out of their control—and the control of their care team—then they are better able to process the unexpected when it occurs. The patient's story I just told you is an example of a situation in which she could have processed the birth very differently than she did. Because she was open and flexible during the process, she was able to accept the things that she could not control and focus on the fact that she felt well cared for, was a part of the decision-making process, and had a good outcome for both her and her baby.

> **It wasn't the birth she wanted, but it was the birth she needed.**

I've already mentioned cesarean births, but it's worth explaining the procedure in more detail here, because the birth experience is very different from a vaginal birth. You may have a planned cesarean birth, or it may be unplanned, with the decision being made during labor. Either way, it is always important to know what to anticipate when you are having a cesarean birth so that the experience is less scary. Your provider may go into detail about the procedure, or they may discuss the basics of the risks, benefits, and alternatives to a cesarean birth. Either way, you should always feel empowered to ask all the questions you have and feel that you still have some agency over how the birth will unfold, even if you give birth in the operating room.

THE REALITY OF C-SECTIONS

Cesarean sections are the most common major abdominal surgery, but most people are completely unprepared for the possibility of having a cesarean birth. In my work with postpartum depression and birth trauma, many patients come to me feeling shocked, traumatized, and depressed after their unplanned C-sections. They are reeling from the experience and often say that they never want to have another baby. Once, a patient came for her two-week postoperative visit, and when I asked her to lie down so I could look at her incision to ensure it was healing properly, she started crying. She had not looked at or even touched her incision. She was still in denial about what had happened to her body and felt completely disfigured by the procedure. When I spoke to her more about it, I learned that her C-section had not been an emergency nor did she have any complications from the surgery. She and her baby were healthy, and the baby did not have to go to the NICU. She had been pushing, but the baby got stuck in the pelvis in such a position that she could not fit through the birth canal, which is called an arrest of descent. Although everything had gone as smoothly as possible, the fact that she was totally unprepared for the possibility of a cesarean birth had left her scarred in more ways than one.

Most people that I care for during pregnancy discuss their birth plan at some point. Some ask about the C-section rates of my practice, and a few ask for an elective scheduled C-section. However, I have never been asked by a patient what I think their individual C-section risk is. This is a hard topic to broach by obstetricians, as we are living during a time in our culture when there is a push for "natural" delivery, which means different things to different people. Many women have shared stories on social media about doctors being aggressive, forcing them into a C-section, and/or not centering their desires. This has created a difficult balance. I want to talk to my patients more about C-sections so that they are prepared for that possibility, but I do not want them to get the impression that I am overly prone to taking my patients to the operating room.

According to Centers for Disease Control birth data from 2019, approximately 30 percent of babies in the United States are born via cesarean section.[1] Of women who are having their first baby and thirty-seven or more weeks at time of birth with a singleton (no multiples) whose head is presenting in the pelvis, approximately 25 percent will have a C-section. A 2018 study in Texas examined risk factors for C-section among a cohort of such women and found that the greatest risk factor for C-section was obesity. Other risk factors such as diabetes, hypertension, preeclampsia, and IVF pregnancy also contributed to a higher rate of C-section. Another important factor shown to increase the risk of C-section was age: women forty years of age and older had a C-section rate of 50 percent. Racial disparities were also noted, with 33 percent of non-Hispanic black women having C-sections, compared with only 25 percent of non-Hispanic white women. Nearly 50 percent of women who had C-sections had at least one maternal risk factor. Black non-Hispanic women had the highest rate of associated risk factors, with 54 percent having at least one risk factor. The greater the number of risk factors, the higher the rate of C-section. Women with no risk factors had a 20 percent risk of C-section, whereas women with three risk factors had a 54 percent chance of C-section.[2]

I am not talking about the risk of C-section to scare moms-to-be nor am I talking about it to justify doing C-sections. When I am on call, I am in the hospital for the full twenty-four hours, so as I tell my patients, it doesn't matter to me whether you deliver at 2:00 p.m. or 2:00 a.m. I will be there no matter what time you give birth. I am not in a rush. I also follow the guidelines from the American College of Obstetricians and Gynecologists and recommend C-sections only for failed induction, arrest of dilation, or arrest of descent when my patients meet the criteria, as long as there is no sign of fetal distress or a maternal reason to move to C-section earlier.

We know from studying patient-reported experience measures (PREM scores) that patients are most likely to be unhappy with their experience when it does not match their expectations. If your preference is a vaginal delivery, you can plan and prepare for that as much as possible and still not get your desired outcome, as with everything else in parenthood. I want birthing people to understand that any time you are delivering a baby, there's a chance that you may need a cesarean birth. I want birthing people and their support systems to understand what happens when they have a C-section so that they can be prepared if their doctor or midwife recommends one for any reason. It is so much better to learn about what happens during a C-section and to process that information before you are heading to the operating room.

THE RISKS OF C-SECTION

Before surgery, your doctor will discuss the risks of having a C-section with you. It can sound scary, but we are morally and legally obligated to discuss even the remote risks with you prior to obtaining your informed consent. These risks include pain, bleeding, infection, damage to surrounding organs such as your uterus, bladder, and bowel, the need for a hysterectomy (removal of your uterus), blood transfusion, and the risk of permanent injury or death to the birth parent and baby. Some patients are at higher risk for different complications. You can ask your doctor about your specific situation. For instance, being in labor for a long time, having fibroids, and having a history of prior abdominal surgery put you at increased risk for bleeding. Obesity, diabetes, intraamniotic infections during labor, and emergency surgery, for which there is no time for a thorough abdominal skin prep (with a sterilizing solution to decrease infection from skin bacteria), put you at increased risk for infection. Prior abdominal surgery and emergency C-sections put you at higher risk for damage to surrounding organs.

WHAT TO EXPECT DURING A C-SECTION

Whether planned or unplanned, any non-emergency cesarean birth can still be a calm experience, and your care team can talk you through it every step of the way. Many people are under the impression that any unscheduled cesarean section is an emergency—this is not true. Very few cesarean births are considered true emergencies, in which we rush to the operating room with the goal of getting the baby out within one minute of making the skin incision because every minute counts for the baby's or birth parent's outcome.

Operating rooms themselves can seem scary, as they are very bright, often cold, sterile environments with a lot of people who have their heads and mouths covered. If you have never been in an OR before, it can feel foreign and uncomfortable. When you enter the OR, everyone should introduce themselves to you. Some of the people you will already know from your care outside of the operating room; they will just look different once their hair and mouths are covered. I always ask my patients if they would like to listen to music while they are prepped for the surgery. We can also keep it on during the surgery, as long as the anesthesiology team is okay with it and we can all communicate effectively. I also have had patients who wanted to mentally remove themselves from the OR, so they wore headphones during the surgery to help with their anxiety. Music can have a calming influence and change your mindset in a scary situation, so you can always prepare playlists for labor and birth, including songs that you may want to listen to in the operating room.

If you have not been in labor, you will walk into the operating room. If you have been in labor, you will be taken in on the labor bed and then transferred to the operating room bed. Initially, once you enter the operating room, your baby will be placed back on the monitor, your blood pressure will be checked, and little stickers that monitor your heart will be placed on your upper body. An IV will be placed if you do not already have one. Sometimes a second IV is placed if the anesthesiologist and obstetrician think you have a higher risk of excessive bleeding so they are prepared in case you need a blood transfusion. At some point, spontaneous compression devices will be put around your lower legs, which fill with air intermittently to maintain blood flow and prevent blood clots.

A cesarean section is typically done with regional anesthesia, such as an epidural, spinal, or both. If you have been in labor and already have an epidural, then that is used and a stronger dose of medication is given for the surgery. If you have not been in labor, either a spinal or a combined spinal/epidural is performed. If there is an emergency and there is no time for regional anesthesia, if the epidural is not working well enough to achieve adequate anesthesia, or if a patient has a medical condition for which regional anesthesia is not an option, general anesthesia is used and the patient is intubated and asleep for the surgery. With regional anesthesia, it is very common to experience shaking, nausea, low blood pressure, and to feel very cold. When my labor epidural was dosed for my first C-section, I felt as if my lower body had been dumped into ice-cold water and I was shaking uncontrollably.

Once you have the appropriate anesthesia in place, you will have a catheter inserted into your bladder if you did not already have one in labor. If your cervix has dilated, your vagina may be cleaned to help prevent bacteria from getting into the uterus and abdomen and causing an infection after your surgery. A sticky pad called a grounding pad will be placed on your thigh. This provides a place for the electrical current from the cautery, or the device that stops bleeding, to flow out of your body. Finally, you will be strapped onto the bed with a belt placed across your thighs so that you can't fall during the surgery. The anesthesiology team may use either something sharp or cold to test that your anesthesia is working effectively and will let your obstetrician know when we are ready for the surgery.

Your abdomen will then be cleaned or "prepped," as we call it in the OR, with a solution meant to decrease your risk of infection by killing the bacteria that naturally grow on your skin. Your doctors will then perform what is called a "time-out," which is a safety check immediately before surgery to ensure that we have the right patient, the right procedure, and are aware of any risk factors for the surgery. The doctors will "test" the anesthesia by pinching your belly where you should be numb so that we are 100 percent sure that the anesthesia level is adequate for your surgery.

A cesarean section involves delivery of the baby through an abdominal incision. Most of the time it is a small incision, approximately 12 centimeters (or less than 5 inches), across the lower abdomen below the bikini line. Occasionally, the incision is made vertically from around the belly button to the pubic bone if a lower abdominal incision seems unsafe for birth parent and baby. If you are not asleep for your surgery, you will know what is going on; you will hear everyone talking in the room and feel touching, pressure, and pulling. You will not feel anything sharp if the anesthesia was tested and found to be adequate. From the start of the surgery until the baby is out typically takes only a few minutes for a first C-section. If you have had prior C-sections or other surgery on your abdomen, you may have scar tissue, so the procedure will take longer. Scar tissue can obscure the natural delineation between organs and tissues, and the surgeon must safely navigate this to get to the uterus without damaging anything else. Refer to the illustration in figure 5.1 for an idea of where the incision is usually made.

When making the incision, your surgeon must cut through several layers to get to your baby:

1. skin
2. subcutaneous adipose, the fat below the skin, which everyone has to some extent
3. fascia, the strong layer that holds everything in your abdominal cavity inside (The muscles under the fascia are separated; they are not cut unless you have a lot of prior scar tissue.)
4. peritoneum, a thin layer lining your entire abdomen and pelvis, which is filled with fluid that coats your internal organs as they move around inside of you
5. uterus

When your baby is born, you will feel a lot of pressure as the baby is guided through the incision (see figure 5.2). If you or your partner want to watch the birth, the anesthesiologist can move the drapes so that you can see the baby lifted up as they enter the world. I always encourage this; it can help provide the same experience as that of first seeing your baby during a vaginal birth even though you are in the OR. Despite what you might have heard (a surprisingly large number of people have been misinformed), you will *not* see your uterus or other internal organs—they all stay inside—you see only your baby and your belly. However, they will be covered in fluids including blood just like in a vaginal birth.

The baby is handed off to a nurse or pediatrician for evaluation, because sometimes babies get fluid in their lungs if they aren't squeezed through the birth canal. Babies that are premature or were stressed may need extra resuscitation from the pediatricians to help them breathe and transition to the outside world. There are different protocols in every hospital for whether the baby, once cleared by the pediatricians,

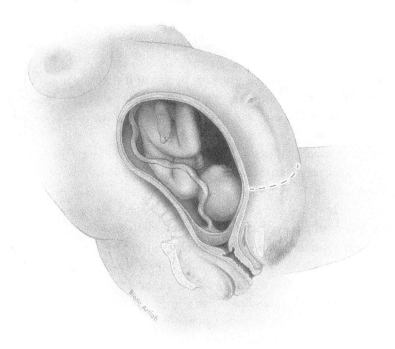

Figure 5.1. C-Section Incision. *Biotic Artlab, 2024*

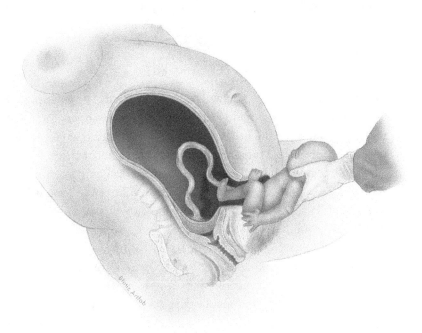

Figure 5.2. C-Section Birth. *Biotic Artlab, 2024*

can go to the birth parent's support person or if the baby needs to be monitored in the warmer. This typically depends on staffing; someone must supervise the baby and the support person if the baby is not left in the warmer.

After the baby is delivered, the surgeons close the layers they had to open to deliver your baby. Interestingly, although the closure of certain layers such as the fascia is critical, research has shown not every layer needs to be closed (for example, the peritoneum). However, surgeons often have different practices and opinions about which layers they typically close based on their training and experience. This part of the surgery typically takes much longer than it took to make the incision. This is because we want to make sure everything goes back the way we found it! Depending on staffing in the operating room, once the baby is evaluated you may be able to have the baby skin-to-skin while the surgery is being finished. This may be delayed until you are moved to the recovery room if there is not an extra staff person in the room to make sure the baby is safely supported. You will be unable to reposition yourself or hold the baby with your arms, because they are extended so the anesthesiologist can access your IVs.

AFTER SURGERY

When you leave the OR, you will be taken to the recovery room. This is where you are monitored closely for the first few hours to ensure that your vital signs and urine output are normal and that you do not have any concerning symptoms. You will have frequent checks by the labor and delivery team to make sure your uterus is staying firm and your lochia (vaginal bleeding) is not too heavy. Afterward, you will be transferred to a postpartum room where you will stay until you are discharged from the hospital.

You may be put on blood thinners to help prevent blood clots. This is a relatively common practice and means that you will have some extra bruising on your abdomen. You may also have a very large dressing over your incision for the first couple of days. Don't worry; your incision is not as big as the bandage! You may have an epidural in place initially for pain control or you may receive intravenous and oral pain medications. There are different protocols at every hospital. You will be woken up a lot overnight so the nurse can check on you and give you medication. Most importantly, you will feel like you had major surgery.

Once your anesthesia wears off, you'll switch to oral plus intravenous medications for breakthrough pain. If you had a spinal (planned C-section) or a dense epidural (placed during labor or when it was determined that you needed a C-section) for the surgery, you usually start to feel more pain within the first hour or so after surgery. Some hospitals leave the epidural in for the first day or so after delivery, or they may give you a percutaneous anesthesia pain pump to help with the immediate pain. Some facilities don't have the resources to provide these services, which require even more oversight and monitoring than oral and intermittent IV medications, so you're immediately switched to as-needed pain control. The first few days are the worst, but it does get better! Having realistic expectations is so helpful, so remind your friends and family that it is not "just a C-section" and that you'll need some extra support and attention while you recover.

Although C-sections are the most common abdominal surgery, they are still major abdominal surgery. For those who are considering an elective C-section or who are in labor but just want to "get it over with," please remember to weigh the risks of major abdominal surgery and the necessary recovery time against your other options before making this decision. However, no one should feel ashamed or judged for having a C-section, no matter whether it was elective or necessary due to labor complications. The American College of Obstetricians and Gynecologists states that it is reasonable for any birthing person to request an elective C-section and after discussing all of the options, risks, and benefits. I always make sure to let my patients know that I support them in their decision. And no matter how your baby comes into the world, you still created, nourished, and delivered a new human being, so you should never feel ashamed or like a failure if you do not have a "natural" birth!

SIX

WHAT HAPPENS AFTER THE BABY IS OUT?

The immediate events after delivery vary depending on the type of birth you had and any complicating factors, such as a preterm birth or a hemorrhage. In this chapter, I discuss the basics of what to expect after the baby has been born. This includes the wide range of feelings you may experience when you first meet your baby, the delivery of the placenta (or afterbirth), and what is involved in the vaginal repair or abdominal closure after C-section. I've often heard questions such as "How many sutures are you using down there?" and "Do you really have to press on my belly now?" This chapter explains all the necessary postpartum steps your care team takes immediately postpartum and the reasons behind them, which may not be verbally relayed to you.

It may seem like once the baby is born, the hard work is over and you should be able to simply relax and get to know your new family member. However, there are still a few more things to take care of before the birth experience is complete. What comes next depends on whether you have had a vaginal birth or C-section.

AFTER A VAGINAL BIRTH

If you gave birth vaginally, the baby can go skin-to-skin immediately unless there is concern that the baby needs resuscitation or extra support transitioning to post-uterine life. Sometimes this is anticipated in advance, such as when a baby is born preterm or with a known complication, and sometimes it happens with a healthy, full-term infant. If the baby needs extra support transitioning, labor and delivery nurses (and possibly pediatric team members—typically specialists from the NICU), will be present at the time of delivery or called as soon as it becomes apparent that more assistance and support is required. If this happens, the baby is often taken to the warmer so that the team has everything they need to easily resuscitate the baby. This can include warm blankets to dry the baby, a bulb suction to clear secretions, supplemental oxygen, and the supplies necessary to give fluids, medications, and intubate in more extreme situations. Luckily, more extensive resuscitation is rarely necessary and occurs most often in very preterm babies or babies with known congenital anomalies or genetic conditions where the likelihood of intubation is known ahead of time.

Once the baby is delivered and the umbilical cord has been cut, the provider collects cord blood to check the baby's blood type and often arterial and venous blood gases from the umbilical cord. These cord gases are helpful when the baby has low APGAR scores (the quick evaluation your baby receives after birth) or when the team needs to determine whether there is evidence of decreased oxygen to the baby's brain in order to monitor and treat the baby appropriately. Many hospitals routinely collect cord blood gases for every baby—just in case—so if your provider collects these, it does not mean they are concerned about your baby.

What happens after this may vary. Sometimes the provider waits for spontaneous separation of the placenta, and sometimes they actively pull on the umbilical cord and massage the uterus to expedite the separation of the placenta from the wall of the uterus. If left alone, the placenta naturally separates within thirty minutes after delivery and comes out of the vagina on its own. If thirty minutes have passed and the placenta has not yet made its appearance, then the provider must determine whether it has separated but remains inside the uterus or if it is still adhered to the uterus, called a retained placenta. If the placenta is retained, extra steps to help separate the placenta from the wall of the uterus may be required. This may involve manual removal by putting their hand inside your uterus to separate the placenta or a procedure called a dilation and curettage (D&C) to surgically remove the placenta in the operating room. These procedures are very uncomfortable, so pain medication through the IV or epidural should be given prior to help make the

procedure more tolerable. It is important that the placenta fully separates and is expelled from your uterus so that you do not develop
excessive bleeding or an infection. A truly retained placenta is rare and
can be associated with something called a placenta accreta, when the
placenta has grown too deeply into the wall of the uterus. This is a rare
but serious complication that is mostly found in people who have had
prior C-sections or fibroids removed and the placenta implants over
the old scar inside the uterus.

Once the placenta has been delivered, the uterus is massaged to
help it begin to contract. Your uterus will still be enlarged from its
original size immediately after delivery. It will shrink to its typical
size by the six-week postpartum mark. Pitocin is often routinely given
to help the uterus contract and to decrease the risks of bleeding after
delivery. It is normal to lose some blood with delivery, no matter how
you give birth. This is why your blood volume expanded significantly
during the third trimester; your body was preparing for the inevitable
loss of some blood volume at the time of giving birth. Vaginal births
typically have a blood loss of 500 milliliters (slightly more than 2 cups)
or less. However, if there is a hemorrhage, the bleeding can be greater.
Physicians and other delivering providers are notorious for underesti-
mating blood loss. This means that, historically, some birthing people
were losing more blood than we accounted for. Due to this, many
hospitals have started weighing the sponges used during delivery and
using drapes that collect the fluids from delivery to better judge. We
also closely monitor the birthing person for symptoms of anemia.
This can be tricky as young, healthy people can compensate a lot, not
showing any signs or experiencing symptoms until their anemia drops
to a critical level. It is always important to tell your provider if you
start to feel lightheaded, dizzy, very weak, or "out of it" or if you feel
chest pain, as if your heart is racing, or short of breath.

If your provider is concerned about a hemorrhage, they will take
extra steps, such as continued uterine massage, extra medications to
help the uterus to contract, additional IV fluids, and an abdominal
ultrasound to check for tissues from the placenta or amniotic membranes left inside your uterus. They will look very closely inside the
vagina and at the cervix to make sure there is not a tear deep inside. If

these steps fail to stop the bleeding, sometimes a special device is used to help tamponade (or to stop via compression) the bleeding. Occasionally patients have to go to the OR to get the bleeding controlled.

Hemorrhage can occur in anyone, even without any noted risk factor; however, there are many risk factors, most commonly:

- history of hemorrhages
- a large baby
- a long labor
- fibroids
- grand multiparity (you have had five or more births before)

The more risk factors you have, the higher the risk for heavier bleeding.

Blood loss typically occurs during delivery or immediately after, but there are also times when someone has a delayed hemorrhage, which can occur hours or days later. Someone might also have slow, persistent bleeding that eventually adds up to a large amount (heavier than normal lochia after birth or even internal oozing after a C-section).

Even if you do not have extra bleeding, the nursing team will be doing frequent checks—called fundal checks—in which they feel the top of your uterus, which should be around the height of your umbilicus, or belly button, postpartum. They press on it (uterine massage) to check how much bleeding comes out of your vagina when they press and to make sure that the uterus feels firm and is not deviated off to the side. This assessment is done to ensure that the uterus is not filling up with blood clots that have not yet come out. Having your abdomen pressed and massaged aggressively is not comfortable, but it is part of the standard postpartum care and helps us to pick up on any concealed bleeding as soon as possible. As I mentioned before, people experiencing a hemorrhage often will not feel symptomatic until their blood count gets very low, at which point it can be harder to correct quickly. The sooner we note any signs of hemorrhage, the better.

If you had tearing during your delivery, the provider will place sutures to stop the bleeding and bring the tissues back together. Tearing is most common on the perineum, or the tissue between the vagina and rectum. Before suturing, your provider should make sure you have adequate pain control, which may be accomplished with the epidural or with local numbing medication such as lidocaine. With either, you may feel touch, pulling, and pressure, but you should not feel sharp pain. Let your provider know if your pain is not controlled so they can get more anesthesia. All of the sutures used to repair tearing with delivery are absorbable, so they never need to be removed. They will dissolve naturally over time. Depending on the location and extent of the tearing, your provider may need an assistant to help with the repair. Stitching in such a delicate area takes careful maneuvering and patience, so the repair can take a while. I have often had patients ask how many sutures I am using, concerned that the tearing must be really bad because it is taking so long. I always explain to patients what kind of tear they have and what I am doing. I also tell them that the repair often feels like it is taking a long time even when the tear is minor.

If you had an epidural with delivery, you need to be able to get up and walk to the restroom prior to going to the postpartum unit, which will be in a separate part of the hospital from labor and delivery. It may be a little while before you feel your legs and have the strength to move. If you had a urinary catheter in your bladder with the epidural, it would have been removed prior to the delivery of the baby, but you still may feel some discomfort or pressure in your urethra (where you urinate from) from the catheter having been there. It is important that you are able to pee after giving birth, because this means that you have regained function of your bladder muscles and can empty your bladder. If the bladder fills up too much, there is a risk that the uterus cannot contract well, since the bladder sits on top of the lower part of the uterus, and that increases the risk for bleeding. We also want to make sure that you are emptying your bladder often, because you get a lot of fluids during labor and if your bladder becomes overly distended, it can rupture. Occasionally, someone cannot pee easily, due to the stress and pressure of the baby's head on the urethra and bladder during pushing, as well as the effects of the anesthesia. If this is the case, a urinary catheter will need to be placed to drain the bladder.

After a few hours of monitoring, you will be transferred to the postpartum floor, which is a different area than where you gave birth. If you had any complications, such as a hemorrhage, you may be monitored a little longer on labor and delivery, since there is typically a higher nurse-to-patient ratio and you can be watched closely.

AFTER A CESAREAN BIRTH

The time from the start of the surgery to when your baby is born is typically quick compared to the time from the birth until the surgery is complete. If you have a stat, or emergency C-section, it may be a mere minute or two from the initial skin incision until your baby is delivered. For a routine first C-section with no prior abdominal surgery, I tell my patients to anticipate forty-five minutes to an hour from start to finish. If you have had prior C-sections or other abdominal surgeries, the timing can vary greatly depending on the amount of scar tissue in your abdomen. The more prior surgeries you have had, the higher the likelihood of scar tissue, which takes more time to safely get into your abdomen and deliver the baby. It takes longer closing everything up, even when there aren't complications, because we have to close the layers of your uterus and fascia properly and ensure there is no oozing or bleeding before it is safe to close your abdomen.

When you have a cesarean birth, the umbilical cord is cut on the sterile operating field, so having your support person cut the umbilical cord as with a vaginal birth is not typically an option. Delayed cord clamping is an option, however, as long as the birth parent and baby are both stable. The baby is then routinely taken to the warmer immediately to make sure there is no fluid in their lungs and to do any additional resuscitation. This is because, with a cesarean birth, the baby is not squeezed through the birth canal, which clears fluids from their mouth and lungs, and they need some suctioning and additional respiratory support to clear and open their lungs. Once the baby has been evaluated and is deemed to be stable, they may be handed to the support person or go skin-to-skin on the birth parent. This often depends on how awake and alert the birth parent is, as well as the ability of a staff person (typically a nurse) to closely monitor the baby while they are with the birth parent and/or support person and also performing necessary tasks required of them in the OR. This is something to ask your care team prior to going to the OR so that you understand what to expect after the birth.

Once your surgery is complete, the support person will be escorted from the OR, the surgical drapes will be removed, and you will be cleaned, a dressing placed over your incision (which often includes a big piece of tape much larger than your actual incision), and transferred to a recovery bed to leave the OR. Just as with a vaginal birth, you will have a uterine massage prior to leaving the OR and again regularly while in the recovery room to make sure your uterus is firm and your bleeding is not concerning. You will also still have an IV hooked up and be very numb from your chest down for a while after surgery. You may be nauseous due to the medication given by the anesthesiologists as well as your abdomen being open and your uterus being manipulated, which can affect your bowels as well.

In the recovery area, your nurse will check on you, frequently monitoring your vital signs (blood pressure, heart rate, oxygen saturation levels) as well as the amount of urine you are making. You will have a foley catheter in your bladder for the first night postpartum until you are able to move around to get to the bathroom and pee.

During this time, you may be exhausted, you may be nauseous, you may be starving, you may be super excited, or you may be ready to fall asleep. You will definitely not get good rest in the recovery area, as the goal of the postsurgical recovery area is close observation by the clinical team, so your nurse, the anesthesiology team, and your obstetric practitioners will be in the room frequently to make sure you are stable. After a few hours, if everything looks good and you do not have any additional complications for which you need to be monitored closely, you will be transferred to the postpartum unit.

MEETING YOUR BABY FOR THE FIRST TIME

After giving birth, one of the most important introductions of your life will occur. You will meet your new baby. Whether your first or your fifth baby, this is always a pivotal experience. There's no way to anticipate what emotions you might feel once your baby delivers. The movies and books often tell us to expect an instantaneous bond, an overwhelming feeling of love and joy—and that might happen. But it's also perfectly normal to feel other emotions, too. If you feel like you are looking at an alien rather than feeling immediate and unconditional love, you are not alone. This does not mean you are a bad parent. I looked at both of my babies with more of a sense of curiosity and awe that the full little human in front of me had just been inside of me. I never felt that I "recognized" them immediately—for one thing, they come out scrunched and covered in fluids, including blood, amniotic fluid, and vernix, a creamy protective barrier like a lotion, which coats a baby's skin inside the uterus. If they came out vaginally, they often have swelling and molding of the head that takes days or weeks to resolve. I never had a preconceived idea about what my baby's face would look like, so it was kind of like going on a blind date with someone you had already committed to marrying.

If you do immediately fall in love with your baby, that's wonderful—and yet you may still want to get as far away from them as possible at times during the coming weeks and months. They also will continue to rapidly change over the first few days and weeks as they adjust to life outside of the uterus. Even the shape of their head and nose changes once they are no longer squished inside! With both of my babies, I felt an attachment in the sense that I was responsible for them, but I did not feel an immediate and intense sense of joy like I expected. It was more a sense of shock and awe that—*holy shit!*—that little human was just inside of me and now there is a completely separate being to take care of. It can be terrifying to think, *I am responsible for making sure they survive and thrive in this crazy world.* I had to get to know my babies in those first days and weeks, and the love grew slowly over time.

All feelings are valid in the aftermath of this life-changing event, and it has absolutely no bearing on your qualification as a parent.

No matter what your initial impression is of your baby, it is okay. All feelings are valid in the aftermath of this life-changing event, and it has absolutely no bearing on your qualification as a parent.

SKIN-TO-SKIN AND LATCHING

The goal is to get the baby skin-to-skin within the first hour. This practice impacts the infant's short- and long-term health, regulation of their vitals, and also promotes bonding. If the birth parent is unable to perform skin-to-skin within the first hour, the partner or another support person can place the baby skin-to-skin, which promotes these benefits for the baby as well. If your baby goes to the NICU, the team will let you know when they can safely be moved for skin-to-skin. Even when it cannot be done immediately after birth, skin-to-skin offers many short- and long-term benefits to babies who start their lives in the NICU, no matter when they are able to achieve skin-to-skin.

For parents who plan to breastfeed or chestfeed, latching on ideally occurs within the first two hours of life. Colostrum—the nutrient-packed form of breast milk that first comes in after birth—can be expressed from the breasts. Although smaller in volume than the milk once it comes in with letdown (typically two to five days after birth), colostrum is rich in calories and can provide your baby with all of the nutrients and hydration they require until your milk comes in. If your baby goes to the NICU or if you are unable to breastfeed/chestfeed within the first few hours for other reasons, the baby can be given formula or, in some places, donor milk until you are able to breastfeed. You can also pump colostrum and later breast milk if your baby is in the NICU.

You may feel the need to constantly have your baby within your sight and to monitor their every action. You may feel exhausted and just want the nurse to take them to the nursery or have your partner hold them so you can get some rest. Your partner or support people will also be going through their own intense emotions and may not feel prepared or ready to hold such a fragile little being. The whole family will adjust and get to know the new baby at their own pace, so try your best not to place expectations on yourself or anyone else. How you bond and form attachments and a loving relationship with your baby may be different from what your friends have told you about their experiences, and that is okay. Just take it day by day.

Extract as much comfort and knowledge about caring for your newborn as you can before you are discharged from the hospital. In the next chapter, I discuss the basic things to expect during your postpartum hospital stay and provide some tips on how to best get your needs met during those few days that you have professionals around to help you.

SEVEN

THE POSTDELIVERY HOSPITAL STAY

The primary objective has been accomplished: you have now birthed your baby! Physically and mentally, there's a lot to process in the immediate aftermath of bringing life into the world. You haven't only birthed a baby. You have also undergone changes to your own identity and physicality. If you had a hospital birth, you'll be staying at least twenty-four hours after a vaginal birth and at least forty-eight hours after a cesarean birth. This chapter describes all the basics that happen during this time, including the endless interruptions, wake ups, and check-ins from your care team. It also gives you some pro tips for how to make sure you get some much-needed rest and recovery before going home with your new baby. I also discuss the surprising range of emotions that you may not have expected to encounter. Finally, I encourage you to advocate for yourself when it comes to getting support from your nurses, lactation consultant, and setting boundaries for visitors. If you feel judged or dismissed, I want you to feel empowered to speak up to get the best care and support possible. You deserve it.

RECOVERING AFTER VAGINAL BIRTH

Once you have given birth, all you will want to do is say hi to your new baby, recover, and sleep (and not necessarily in that order). But you have a busy twenty-four to forty-eight hours ahead before it may be time to leave the hospital. The baby may be on you, in the warmer, or possibly even in the NICU if born early or requiring additional support. Your OB provider may be putting some sutures in your perineum or vagina if you had tearing with your birth. Your nurse will be buzzing around you, making sure your vital signs and your bleeding are okay, pressing on your uterus to make sure it is firm, and checking on the baby. You may also be getting medications through your IV and, occasionally, shots in your thigh to help with bleeding if it is heavier than normal. The good news is that if everything looks good, you will be able to have a nice full meal, perhaps the first in a while if you had a long labor.

Typically, you will spend a few hours on labor and delivery to make sure your bleeding is normal and that you are able to walk to the bathroom to pee before you are transferred to the postpartum floor. Depending on your hospital and the staffing, the baby may room with you or go to the nursery for stretches of time. If you need to rest and recover, it is always okay to ask your nurse to take the baby to the nursery. Sometimes new parents are met with resistance to this, especially in baby friendly hospitals where the goal is to keep the baby with the parents for as much of the stay as possible; however, babies have been accidentally dropped or suffocated when the birth parent is so exhausted that they fell asleep while holding the baby. Do not feel guilty asking someone to take the baby if it will help you get some much-needed sleep and recovery time. The nurses who work on postpartum and in the nursery love babies— they will always take excellent care of them when they are out of your sight. (Many times I have witnessed them talking sweetly to these little ones and walking around, cuddling them in their arms. They really love babies!)

Once you are transferred to a postpartum room, you will have a new care team, which includes your nurse and often a technician who may draw your blood or take your vitals, as well as a lactation consultant to help you learn how to breastfeed/chestfeed, pump, and hand express, depending on your feeding goals. If you are exclusively formula feeding, your team will know this from the time of your admission. Often new parents feel guilty for formula feeding, but this is a very personal decision, and no matter your reason for making this choice, you can still bond with your baby, perform skin-to-skin, and give them all the proper nutrition they need to grow and thrive. You can include your feeding preferences in your birth plan and even create a full feeding plan in advance that states the order of your feeding preferences and how you plan to feed throughout the day and night. The Fed Is Best Foundation has excellent resources to help you create an evidence-based feeding plan for your baby.[1]

On the postpartum floor, you will still get frequent check-ins from your nurse and the other support staff. They will be checking your vital signs, your uterus, and your pads to make sure there are no concerning signs such as high or low blood pressure or heavy bleeding. They will also ask if you are peeing and if you have been passing gas or pooping. They may place a "hat" in the toilet bowl (something to catch the urine and blood) so they can directly visualize the amount of blood that comes out from your vagina into the toilet. They will also ask you to rate your pain on a scale of one to ten and ask how you feel when you get up to walk to the restroom or around the postpartum floor.

RECOVERING AFTER CESAREAN BIRTH

You're typically kept in the hospital for two to four days after the surgery. You shouldn't be discharged until your pain is controlled with oral medications. This doesn't mean that you'll feel great. In fact, you won't be able to do much more than walk to the bathroom. But if getting out of bed is impossible without severe pain, make sure your nurses and doctors know before they send you home, and if something doesn't feel right and you feel ignored or your symptoms dismissed, enlist your support system to advocate for you.

Every time you get up and put pressure on your abdominal muscles, you'll feel the sharp pain of having had surgery. Even at rest, you'll feel soreness and inflammation. Using an abdominal binder or bracing with a pillow every time you have to cough or sneeze can help. Although binders don't help with the healing process, they often help birth parents feel that their internal organs are held in. This also helps them feel more comfortable, especially during the initial weeks of healing, when the abdominal muscles are very relaxed and everything internally feels out of place. I tell my patients that the first few weeks are the worst and then, hopefully, the pain has improved enough that you can take longer walks and get out of the house for brief periods of time with or without the baby.

You'll most likely feel much better about one month post-op, although you still won't be completely recovered from surgery. Even if you feel back to your baseline, remember that you still should not be doing anything strenuous or that puts pressure on your abdominal muscles or pelvis until you're cleared by your doctor at your six-week visit. Some people continue with higher pain levels for longer than the first few weeks or go home and then experience excruciating pain. If this happens, reach out to your doctor immediately for reevaluation. You know your body, your own pain tolerance, and your history, and if you feel like something is not right, you should reach out for help and further evaluation.

If you had a C-section, the postpartum course varies based on where you delivered. This is because post-surgery pain management methods vary from place to place. Some use a spinal for anesthesia for scheduled surgeries, so you immediately transition to IV and oral pain management. Some places use a combined spinal/epidural or a dense epidural only if you needed a C-section in labor. They may or may not remove the epidural immediately after surgery. If they leave it in, they can use this for pain management. It's often called a "walking epidural," as the dose is not as heavy as during surgery or labor, so it helps with pain control but does not make you so numb that you cannot walk around. Either way, at some point you will transition to IV and then oral-only pain medication. You cannot be discharged from the hospital until your pain is controlled without IV medication. This does not mean you will not have pain; it just means that you can function and get up and move around (minus strenuous activity) without being in pain severe enough that you ask for stronger pain medication.

Throughout this time, your team also will be checking on the baby and asking about the baby's wet diapers and if they passed stool. The baby will need some basic tests prior to discharge, such as the hearing test and bilirubin test associated with jaundice. A newborn screening panel is frequently done in the hospital to look for rare but serious conditions. These tests vary state by state and the pediatrician monitoring your baby in the hospital can provide more information about the testing done in your state.

REST AND RECOVERY

It is really hard to get any decent rest while in the hospital. You are caring for your brand-new baby while having people checking on you round the clock to assess everything mentioned earlier. You also may be facing a lot of requests from friends and family to visit you and meet the new baby. However, getting as much rest as possible so that you can begin your recovery is very important. Being in the hospital may mean a lot of extra people checking on you; however, these are also people who can help you by watching the baby in the nursery for a few hours so that you can sleep. You also can engage your support team to help with the baby so you can rest. For your physical recovery, make sure you are eating and staying hydrated. If you are breastfeeding or chestfeeding, you will need extra hydration and calories to help support milk production. If you had surgery or a vaginal tear, it is important to eat a lot of protein to help your body rebuild and repair the cut or torn tissues.

Besides feeling empowered to ask your team of doctors, nurses, techs, lactation consultants, and additional hospital support staff for help, I want you to feel empowered to ask your personal support team for anything you need or want them to help you with. Advocate for yourself—know your needs and ask for help. Often, even those who love us very much are unable to anticipate our needs right after delivery, or they may be tempted to focus on the baby more than the birth parent. Let them know how they can be of service to you, whether it is getting you some coffee, running out to get that nipple cream the lactation consultant recommended, or calling the pediatrician to let them know you've delivered and schedule the newborn exam. Sometimes it's just reminding them to check in on how you are feeling and to hold space for you to talk and reflect on your experience.

EMOTIONAL RECOVERY

An often overlooked but very important aspect of your postpartum course is the emotions you feel as you begin to process your experience and understand your new identity as parent to this little infant who has suddenly entered the world. Even if you had the birth experience of your dreams, there is still a lot to process emotionally about giving birth: the way your body looks when you see yourself for the first time in the mirror, the way you feel about your new identity and massive responsibility, the way you feel about your new baby. There may have been parts of your experience that were scary, unexpected, or very different than how you envisioned them.

Even when everything goes as planned, there is still a major, life-altering shift that happens when you give birth. The way Vaishnavi Tallury, occupational therapist and mother of two, explained it to me really resonated and helped me understand and process my emotional responses after giving birth the first time:

> We don't talk about the disruption in your roles and routines and identity. That is what women experience through birth. Pregnancy is a long time. It's nine months and it is a slow and steady progression. Then one day you're pregnant and then the next day you're not, in that period of time called labor and delivery. It's insane. You have this routine, you go to your job, you do your thing, and then, all of a sudden, that stops. Something new starts that you have had really no way of preparing for. And that disruption, that shift in identity, is extremely disorienting.[2]

I recall the postpartum hospital stay after the birth of my first daughter as a surreal, disorienting experience. Intellectually, I fully comprehended that I had just given birth and had a new baby. That was a fact I accepted implicitly. But processing this and incorporating it into what I knew to be true about myself was very hard. I went to my safe space, a place I felt comfortable and a role I knew very well: I went into doctor and caretaker mode. I tried to jump out of bed and do things like I usually would, even though I had just had experienced the physical trauma of a major abdominal surgery. I was not letting myself just sit with the fact that I'd just gone through this overwhelming experience and now had a new identity as a mother. I just wanted to do what I knew how to do best—take care of the needs of others. I had to feed this baby. I had to make sure she was warm and clean and dry. The fact that she was my daughter, I was her mother, and she had just come into the world via a major abdominal surgery that would require a long and painful recovery was not really entering my mind. That processing of my birth experience and my matrescence—the process of becoming a mother—took a long time to understand and integrate.

Our individual birth experiences and our perception of those experiences can vary tremendously, as will our emotions during the immediate postpartum period. But no matter your experience, perception, and emotions, adjusting from being pregnant to not being pregnant and to the drastic changes this causes immediately in your daily routine can be shocking and difficult to process. It's okay to not seamlessly transition to being the new parent you thought you would be. It's okay to feel overwhelmed and scared and not to fall in love with your baby immediately. It's okay to feel so exhausted that you just want to sleep for days and can't even think about the baby. Basically, there are no taboo or shameful feelings surrounding giving birth. If your emotions are extreme and you can't function normally, however, always ask for help from your care team. Severe anxiety, depression, and other more rare but serious mental health conditions can take hold quickly after birth, and we want you to get the help you need before you leave the hospital.

SETTING BOUNDARIES FOR VISITORS

So many birthing parents let themselves be miserable to make other people happy. They will skip a nap and become even more sleep-deprived so that their family who wants to meet the new baby can come and visit as soon as possible. Sometimes, parents don't even know what they need because they've never been in this situation before, so it's easier to listen to others' suggestions than to do the hard work (when they're exhausted!) of figuring out what actually might be best for *them*. I know you want to make your friends and family happy, but do not do it at your own expense. If having them visit and meet the baby helps you feel good, boosts your morale, calms your stress, and alleviates some anxieties, then please encourage them to visit or even ask directly for help. However, if it feels like an obligation that will only add to your stress, anxiety, and inability to rest and recover, then please feel empowered to put your own needs before the needs of everyone else. Your baby needs a healthy parent more than they need to meet your in-laws or friends.

Once you have met all of your immediate postpartum milestones and you are cleared to go home, you will move on to the next phase: postpartum recovery at home. This can be scary and a little daunting, but it also can be very exciting, as you may be impatient to get back home and start the next phase of life in a comfortable environment. I do want to stress that if you feel like something might be wrong that your care team has not yet addressed or seems to minimize (such as pain that is not yet well controlled or dizziness while walking), please advocate for yourself and make sure you have a satisfactory answer regarding your symptoms and a plan in place before discharge. You know your body and you should never leave the hospital if you feel like your care team has not properly addressed your concerns.

If this is your first time as a parent, you may be asking yourself how anyone could trust you to leave the hospital without supervision and care for such a vulnerable little creature as your newborn baby. The secret is that no one ever feels prepared—we all just do it! In the same way, we are never fully prepared for all of the self-care involved in our own recovery. In the next chapter, I discuss the main aspects of your own post-birth recovery that you will be faced with after leaving the hospital. It may seem impossible, but you will start to feel like yourself again over the coming days, weeks, and months. You can do this; you are ready to take on these challenges!

In part II, I delve into some of the major issues people struggle with over and over again during the early postpartum period. So many aspects of this time period simply aren't explored deeply in conversations with health care providers, friends, family, or those on social media who we turn to when we imagine what our life will look like after we bring home a baby. I want to offer you a realistic idea about what to expect and how your idealized vision of postpartum life may drastically differ from what you encounter along your journey. This is not meant to scare you, but rather to prepare you in a supportive way that embraces the messiness and unpredictability of this journey.

Caring for a newborn while also considering the needs of your partner and everyone else you don't want to disappoint is *hard*. You already may be used to putting your needs last. But because you matter, your physical and emotional recovery matter, your ability to fill your own cup matters, and your ability to bond with your new baby matters, these topics deserve open and honest discussion.

PART II

Postpartum

EIGHT

POSTPARTUM RECOVERY

There is pain.

There is bleeding.

There is incontinence (urine, gas, stool—sometimes simultaneously!).

There is breast engorgement, leaking, and pain.

There are massive hormonal shifts.

There is sleep deprivation and exhaustion.

There is love. Lots of love. (As well as many other completely valid emotions!)

The first time I exercised after having my first daughter, I was shocked. I had gone into her birth working out regularly up until my due date. However, when I returned to the gym, I realized I had no core strength. I would have to completely retrain my abdominal muscles. I also was much weaker generally, and my balance was not as good as it had been; my center of gravity had shifted completely from where it had been before giving birth. I felt defeated and humbled that I had lost all of my strength and everything I had worked so hard for before having a baby.

No matter how delivery occurs, birth parents are often surprised by some of the physical symptoms they experience postpartum. I frequently speak to new parents who felt that if they had vaginal births, they'd go home and "bounce back," or quickly return to their prepregnancy bodies. However, even vaginal births require time for healing from tearing, swelling, stretching, hemorrhoids, and the pain that comes along with them. Although the postpartum period lasts the first year of birth, in this chapter I cover the normal spectrum of your postpartum physical recovery during the first six weeks after giving birth and provide some tips for in-the-moment management of these uncomfortable recovery symptoms. The first six weeks, particularly the first two, is the most intense period of physical recovery. I also discuss warning signs for which you should seek help or go to the emergency room. Of course, there is a lot more going on than just physical recovery when you're postpartum, and I cover more about your emotions and mental health in the next chapter.

THE FIRST SIX WEEKS

No matter how you deliver the baby, you'll experience at least some pain, swelling, bleeding, and possibly urinary, fecal, and/or flatal incontinence (this means peeing, pooping, or passing gas without trying, respectively). Many new moms are surprised by the pain they feel and the recovery period required for even a vaginal birth. They assumed delivering vaginally would mean they could quickly and easily get back to their pre-baby physical state. This is all overwhelming, I know, but stay with me! Let's dive into those symptoms more deeply and explore how to manage the discomfort.

Managing Your Pain

You may have bad tearing or minimal to no tearing but still feel like your bottom was destroyed from hours of pushing. You may experience swelling and soreness. You may be scared to look at your vagina and perineum or your abdomen if you had a C-section, as it feels as if nothing will ever be the same again. This feeling of dread and despair often resolves by the six-week mark. Believe it or not, even women who were still really struggling physically a few weeks after delivery typically feel much better by the six-week mark. And if it takes you longer than six weeks, that's okay, too. Remember, no two bodies and no two pregnancies are alike, so be gentle with yourself, just like you are with your newborn. Caring for yourself through the pain and recovery one day at a time is all that you can do.

To help with the pain, I recommend:

- Ice packs on the perineum or over the C-section scar to help reduce swelling and inflammation
- A donut or pillow under your bottom when you sit
- Pain medication: You can alternate between Tylenol (acetaminophen) and Motrin (ibuprofen) around the clock. If you take them at the same time, there will be periods when they're wearing off before your next dose is due.

  You may have been given narcotics, like Percocet or morphine, in the hospital. Use initially if needed; however, if you require frequent doses of narcotics or if the pain is worsening, always speak to your care provider to make sure your level of pain is not an indication of something more serious. Take extra caution if you have a history of substance use disorder.

  Numbing medications—such as Dermoplast if you have swelling, stitches, or hemorrhoids—can provide extra relief from the discomfort.
- A peri-wash bottle is helpful for when you pee if you have any vaginal tearing. When urine hits the raw tissue that's healing, it burns, and you want to splash water on it as soon as possible to help neutralize the acid. You also can buy a bidet attachment for your toilet if you prefer—many brands easily install directly to your toilet without need for a plumber.

Recovering from a Vaginal Birth

The first few weeks of healing may be extremely painful, especially if you had extensive tearing or an episiotomy. New moms are often shocked, because they thought their recovery would be easy if they could avoid a C-section. In more than a decade as a practicing obstetrician, I've cared for many birthing people whose first vaginal birth involved a tear into their rectum and who subsequently opted for an elective cesarean birth with their next baby. They often report that the recovery from the C-section was easier than from the vaginal birth.

Sometimes there is so much pain and swelling that it is hard to sit, walk, or have a bowel movement. (Remember those ice packs, peri-wash bottles, numbing sprays, and pain medications that I mentioned earlier? They come in handy here, too.) Also, make sure your support system is aware that you won't be "bouncing back." They may anticipate that you'll be able to move around and do more and, in reality, you're cringing every time you walk to the bathroom.

If you had a vaginal birth, the way you feel and recover after delivery will be influenced by many factors:

- whether you have had prior vaginal births
- how big your baby was and the position of the baby's head
- the shape of your pelvis
- how long you pushed
- how much tearing you had and where it is located
- if you had an episiotomy
- if you had an operative delivery with vacuum or forceps
- whether you had other complications such as bleeding after delivery (or postpartum hemorrhage)
- your basic underlying physical status and pain tolerance

Some women have no tearing but still suffer from swelling, soreness, and intense tailbone or pubic symphysis pain after delivery. Some women have tears but feel pretty good soon after. There is no right or wrong way to feel after a vaginal birth. Besides the physical trauma, the process of delivering a baby, no matter how lovely or uncomplicated the delivery, is still experienced as trauma for many people. Pushing something the size of a watermelon through a very small tunnel that must stretch immensely to accommodate it—often causing intense pain, tearing, and bleeding—can be scary and traumatic no matter how much you love your baby when it's all over.

Unless you had extensive tearing or complications such as a wound infection or sutures opening up, you'll start to feel better after the first two weeks. You won't feel 100 percent, but walking and sitting will be more tolerable. For others, the extent of their tearing leads to prolonged pain, and they don't feel closer to full recovery until four to six weeks postpartum. Some women still feel pain, pulling, tightness, and soreness at their six-week visit. This can be due to inflammation and scar tissue formation. If this is your case, I highly recommend seeing a pelvic floor physical therapist to help relax the muscles and the scar tissue and desensitize the pain receptors, especially before you consider having intercourse.

Recovering from a Cesarean Birth

A common but extremely dismissive and minimizing phrase I have heard from patients and other obstetric providers is "It's *just* a C-section." Even though cesarean sections are one of the most common surgeries performed every day, they're still major abdominal surgeries. This means that they come with the risks of other major abdominal surgeries, such as hysterectomy or bowel injury, as well as the risks of anesthesia, including severe allergic reactions and cardiac events. Because C-sections involve having your abdomen cut open, a baby removed, and then your abdomen closed again, the very real and intense pain you'll feel after the surgery is nothing to dismiss or minimize.

Caring for thousands of women over more than a decade in various hospital settings, performing their C-sections, and monitoring them as they recovered prepared me for my own unplanned C-section. I understood and respected the surgery and necessary anesthesia for what they were, including all the risks and postpartum struggles that may have come.

Apart from my own experience of having two C-sections, I have been a part of and heard about vastly different birth stories from people who have had C-sections over the years. Many different factors can affect the experience of the surgery and the postoperative recovery.

If you have had prior cesarean sections or other abdominal surgery, your recovery and pain may be worse than with your prior surgery. This is because you may have internal scar tissue, which may require more pulling and dissection to get to the baby and deliver them safely without injuring your surrounding pelvic organs.

If you had a long labor prior to the C-section or an emergency surgery, your recovery may also be more difficult. A long labor is exhausting and may also mean increased blood loss at the delivery because your uterus is also tired and may not contract as easily to stop bleeding once the baby is delivered.

If you have emergency surgery, the time from starting the surgery to delivery of the baby may be as quick as one minute—a lot of pulling and stretching versus slow dissection is done in these cases because every minute counts and could lead to a worse outcome for the baby if your team doesn't act quickly enough. Also, if you didn't have an epidural already when it was determined that you needed emergency surgery, you may be intubated with general anesthesia and wake up in the recovery area with more intense pain without the effects of regional anesthesia (an epidural) to help.

WHAT'S NORMAL AFTER BIRTH?

No matter how you gave birth, there are some physical experiences that are common for all new birth parents.

Bowel Movements

You may not even have had a bowel movement in the hospital before you go home after a vaginal birth or a C-section. No matter how you give birth, it can be scary to have the first bowel movement. Most people who have sutures on the perineum or abdomen are very worried about bearing down to have a bowel movement and risk opening their sutures. I can reassure you that I have never had anyone open up their wound due to a bowel movement, and pooping is not as painful as most people fear it will be. To help make the process less stressful on your body, stay well hydrated, use stool softeners, eat lots of fiber, and take a laxative if needed. If you had a C-section, you should at least pass gas and be able to eat food without getting nauseated or vomiting before you leave the hospital. It's common to still feel bloated and distended as your intestines start to move more regularly after the narcotics and the surgery. Just as after a vaginal birth, a regimen to help prevent constipation and improve your gut motility can be helpful.

Bruising

You may also have bruising and swelling around the incision. When I looked at my belly the first week or so after my surgery, I felt like I had come home from battle. I had deep purple and black bruising due to the hospital-provided blood thinners to prevent blood clots and the stretching of my tissues to deliver my baby. The bruising extended a few inches above my incision down to my labia. My labia were also so swollen from pregnancy and fluids during labor that I felt like my body wasn't my own. It is a common experience to look at your body and feel horrified, traumatized, or as if you don't know yourself anymore.

You'll start to feel more like yourself over time, but it may take a while, so try to practice self-love and self-acceptance in the meantime. As with everything else in life, this too shall pass. One day in the not-so-distant future, you'll look down and see only a thin scar on your abdomen and explain to your toddler that this is where they popped out of mommy's belly. You'll explain to them that you're the hero who put your baby's health above all else and went through a major abdominal surgery so that they could come into the world safely.

Swelling and Fluid Retention

Your body will be carrying a lot of extra fluid after you deliver. This is mainly due to the massive increase in blood volume during pregnancy in preparation for the blood loss that happens with birth. Additionally, liters of fluids are given prior to and during surgery—and even more if you labored prior to surgery. This means you'll inevitably have lots of swelling in your legs and arms after delivery. This fluid buildup in your tissues usually gets absorbed into your bloodstream and is peed out within the first few days after delivery. For some people, the swelling is so severe that it is painful to move and bend their joints or even rest due to the intense pressure on their skin. If this is the case, the doctor may give you medication to help you diurese, or pee, more to clear out the extra fluid quicker.

A lot of new moms are also very surprised by how swollen the labia and perineum can be after delivery. Part of this surprise is that they haven't been able to see their own genitalia for months due to the pregnant belly. The swelling starts before birth as the pressure of the expanding belly decreases blood flow returning to the upper body, leading to swollen legs, labia, hemorrhoids, and varicose veins. Additionally, during labor and pushing, the swelling increases due to the fluids you are given and the pressure from the baby's head sitting on the perineum while pushing. This will improve with time. However, ice packs can be helpful in the initial days. You will mobilize and clear out the extra fluid by peeing it out, especially during the first few weeks after giving birth.

Drainage

If you had a C-section, a little oozing of blood or clear fluid from the incision is common in the first week or so as the skin heals. You can use a cotton pad or gauze over the incision to protect your clothing and to make sure the moisture is pulled away from your skin. If the incision stays moist or wet, an infection of the skin, such as a yeast infection or bacterial infection, increases as well as the risk of the incision opening. A few drops are okay, but if there is a lot of leakage of fluid, call your doctor. It could be a collection of blood or fluid below the skin, or, even more dangerous, an opening in the fascia, the strong layer that holds all your intestines inside the abdomen.

Bleeding

You'll have postpartum bleeding, or lochia, for four to six weeks after delivery, even if you had a cesarean section. The bleeding starts off as a heavy period. There may be some small clots, especially when you first get up in the morning and after breastfeeding/pumping, as the uterus contracts from the oxytocin released with breastfeeding. Once the initial bleeding subsides, you may have irregular spotting or bleeding or no bleeding at all if you breastfeed/pump. As you space out the feedings, you may return to normal periods or you may have no periods until you stop breastfeeding. If you don't breastfeed/pump, then your periods return within the first month or so after the lochia stops. Just remember that you can ovulate even when you breastfeed. You also can start to ovulate regularly postpartum, even if you weren't ovulating regularly prior to pregnancy or had unexplained infertility.

Hemorrhoids

Hemorrhoids are very common during pregnancy. The good news is they improve and often even resolve completely during the initial postpartum period. This is because the uterus and baby are no longer putting pressure on the veins in your pelvis, causing the blood to back up and create hemorrhoids. In the initial postpartum period, you may be dealing with the pain and discomfort of hemorrhoids; however, with patience they rarely require interventions and quietly resolve on their own. The best way to help them to go away is to avoid getting constipated, as the increased pressure when trying to have a bowel movement puts more pressure on the veins of the hemorrhoids. See the earlier section about bowel movements. For pain and itching from hemorrhoids, Preparation H, Dermoplast, and Tucks cooling pads can help.

Incontinence

You may pee yourself. Sexy, I know. It may occur only when you sneeze or cough. Or you may be totally incontinent and randomly leak urine for a little while. If you don't like the huge pads, just buy adult diapers, which work for both urine and blood. You may also pass gas without trying or even have some fecal (stool) incontinence during early postpartum. The vagina and uterus sit between the bladder and rectum. Throughout your whole pregnancy, the weight of the baby not only puts pressure on your pelvic bones and muscles, but also on the support system of the bladder and rectum.

Even if you have a cesarean birth, you can have a weak pelvic floor and incontinence after delivery. If you pushed for a long time, had a large baby, required forceps, or had a third- or fourth-degree perineal tear (one that goes into your rectum), you're at higher risk of incontinence. The good news is that, for most women, it starts to get much better after the first few weeks. By the six-week visit, it has resolved for most new moms. If not, at this point it is reasonable to not only do your Kegels, but also to ask for a referral for pelvic floor physical therapy and a urogynecologist who specializes in female pelvic floor prolapse and incontinence.

I promise this is only temporary and, like I mentioned, the majority of people feel close to their baseline by the six-week mark and are excited to get back to normal activities. This is not the case for everyone, so if you have any concerns about your physical recovery, even if the provider says everything looks normal on the exam, please speak up and make sure you have a good plan if something just isn't feeling right.

WHEN TO CALL THE DOCTOR

If your recovery is moving along, and then you suddenly have more intense pain, bleeding, abnormal discharge, signs of an infection, or what some patients describe as feeling like a stitch popped open, call your provider immediately and go back for an evaluation to make sure the wound is not opening and that you're not getting an infection. Any drainage that looks like pus (typically white or yellow in color) or smells bad is a sign of infection. This may or may not be accompanied by a fever, so don't wait for a fever to develop if you have other symptoms of an infection.

If you had a cesarean birth, it is normal not to be able to see the incision right after your delivery, as the abdominal muscles are stretched and may relax and cover the incision. Checking your incision daily in the mirror may not sound like the most appealing thing to do, but it is important. If you cannot easily see it, then you should have someone else looking at it every day to make sure that there are no warning signs of complications.

If swelling suddenly increases, especially more in one side, such as one leg more than the other, if swelling is red and painful, or if you have symptoms such as shortness of breath, chest pain, heart racing, headaches, or just not feeling well or normal, please call your doctor immediately. This may be a sign of a very serious condition such as a blood clot in your leg, which can travel to your lungs, or high blood pressure or preeclampsia, which can occur after delivery, even if you had normal blood pressure during pregnancy and delivery. Preeclampsia typically involves high blood pressure and can also affect your other major organs, leading to severe and life-threatening conditions such as seizures or strokes.

I know this is a lot, and it sounds scary, but as long as you know what to look out for, then you can confidently go home knowing that your ankles will reappear someday soon, and—unless you have any additional concerning symptoms—this is just a normal part of postpartum recovery!

PRIORITIZING YOURSELF DURING RECOVERY

Sometimes I feel like my primary job is to give my patients permission and to actively encourage them to prioritize themselves during their recovery. From someone who has been there herself and supported countless others along this intense part of their journey, please keep in mind these words of advice I share with my patients and loved ones navigating the early weeks of recovery and new parenthood:

- Be gentle to your body while you're recovering and ask for help/delegate so that you can recover safely from giving birth.
- Your tasks during the early days are limited to healing, sleeping, hydrating, eating, bonding with your baby, and feeding your baby (however you choose to feed your baby).
- Speak to yourself the same way you'd speak to your best friend. You would never speak critically of your best friend's body after they just birthed a baby, but for some reason, we're very harsh toward ourselves and don't give ourselves the same compassion we give to those we love.

Relying on others can leave you feeling frustrated, upset, guilty, or incompetent. These feelings will pass as you regain your autonomy (which you will, I promise!). However, it is so important to learn to ask for help and to explicitly state what you need help with to those around you.

In the next chapters, I explore in more detail other aspects of the early weeks of postpartum life and what it looks like to start getting back to feeling like yourself emotionally and physically. For the early days, just remember, *this too shall pass*. Nothing is permanent, and it does get easier.

NINE

BABY BLUES AND PERINATAL MENTAL HEALTH DISORDERS

Parents-to-be are often so caught up in thinking about how they'll give birth and care for the infant once they go home from the hospital that they often don't prepare themselves for their personal recovery from childbirth and the transition that occurs as they enter parenthood. We ask our friends what the first few weeks were like caring for a new baby, but not what it felt like caring for *themselves* after giving birth. There are intense emotional changes that go along with the physical changes discussed in chapter 8. You may feel a sense of awe and empowerment by what your body just accomplished. That feeling may help you embrace your post-baby body since it has brought life into the world.

However, more often, I hear stories that aren't so positive. Many birth parents are very critical of themselves. The lack of preparation for the reality of birth and postpartum, along with the images we are surrounded with in the media that don't accurately reflect the experience of most birth parents, sets us up for an inability to accept our own experiences. This is important on our journey toward healing as we gain a renewed sense of self—physically, mentally, and emotionally.

There is also often a sense of mourning. Losing yourself and having to figure out who you are as you incorporate being a parent into your identity. This transition, termed "matrescence," is discussed further in later chapters. Your mental and emotional states are highly involved in this transition and can be affected deeply but are often overlooked by everyone around you as the focus tends to be on caring for the new baby much more than caring for the birth parent. Perinatal mental health providers often describe this situation using an analogy of a piece of candy. The birth parent is the wrapper and the baby is the candy—once the enticing piece of candy is unwrapped, the wrapper is tossed aside and forgotten.

In this chapter, I discuss the emotional and mental changes that occur postpartum and warning signs for when baby blues may have tipped over into a clinical mental health disorder such as anxiety or depression. I also provide some resources and support to help guide you and prepare you for this aspect of your postpartum journey. Bringing home a baby is one of the biggest changes you will experience in your life, and learning how much love and responsibility you are capable of feeling can be incredible. However, it also can be extremely intense with other emotions that may dominate, so I want to help you to feel prepared to understand what is normal, when you should get help, and how you can get help.

BABY BLUES

New parents are often taught that baby blues are common, but not exactly what the "baby blues" are or how long they last. This leaves them unprepared for the other symptoms that occur in the immediate postpartum due to the drastic drops in estrogen and progesterone, such as hot flashes and other perimenopause-like symptoms. Understanding what is normal can help you discern the normal emotional changes that occur along with hormonal shifts from the more extreme symptoms of postpartum depression, which is discussed in the next chapter.

Baby blues are extremely prevalent. Approximately 80 percent of birth parents experience baby blues.[1] What we typically imagine when we think of a very "hormonal" new parent is one whose mood shifts from laughing to crying, without knowing why they are crying, only to quickly fluctuate again to a happier state. Baby blues are caused by the sudden rapid shift in hormones after delivery. The placenta produces the majority of estrogen and progesterone during pregnancy, and by the time you give birth, these two hormones are at the highest levels they will ever be in your lifetime. After the placenta is expelled when you give birth, your estrogen and progesterone levels rapidly drop drastically, to one of the lowest levels you will ever experience. It's as if you have shifted into menopause overnight (with accompanying hot flashes, night sweats, and vaginal dryness as an added bonus!). This drop—as well as the drop in cortisol and positive endorphins released when you give birth, which start to fall significantly within the first few hours after birth—leads to your postpartum mood changes. Baby blues occur with these hormonal drops. Often birth parents feel anxious and overwhelmed from the drop in progesterone. They also experience episodes of tearfulness and easily cry, which often occurs suddenly and then stops just as suddenly.

Baby blues are different from postpartum depression, and it is important to be able to recognize the difference. Postpartum depression is discussed in detail later in this chapter, but the major distinction between the two are the onset, duration, and severity of symptoms. Baby blues occur only within the first two weeks postpartum. If symptoms last longer than this or are more severe, you are experiencing more than just baby blues, and it usually does not just "go away" on its own. Postpartum depression also can occur within the first two weeks, as well as its potentially life-threatening extreme versions, postpartum mania and postpartum psychosis, so if your mood swings feel like more than the mild fluctuations described above, tell your partner or another loved one and seek help from a trusted care provider.

When you feel you are experiencing baby blues and you just can't stop crying or change your mood, I recommend doing something to distract yourself. My self-prescribed remedy for my own postpartum baby blues the second time around was *Ted Lasso*. I needed something that was uplifting and that I enjoyed watching during these moments when I felt emotionally overwhelmed and seemed to cry for no reason. Find something that can distract you from whatever triggered the crying spell. It may be nothing at all that really started the shift in emotions, and that's okay, too—anything lighthearted that historically has made you feel good can help pull you out of these intense hormonal responses more quickly.[2]

POSTPARTUM DEPRESSION/PERINATAL
MENTAL HEALTH DISORDERS (PMHDS)

PMHDs are still often lumped into the category of postpartum depression, a very narrow term that encompasses a broad spectrum of mental health disorders and not just the classic depression symptoms. This group of mental health disorders includes anxiety, depression, obsessive compulsive disorders (OCD), panic disorder, post-traumatic stress disorder (PTSD), bipolar disorder, and postpartum psychosis. Perinatal suicide, which is defined as suicide during pregnancy through the first year postpartum, causes more deaths among birth parents than hemorrhage, preeclampsia, or blood clots. If you were unaware of how common, diverse, and severe PMHDs are, you are not alone.[3]

Throughout the COVID-19 pandemic, we learned more than ever the importance of having the support of friends and family in our lives. I have seen so many new parents struggling because their own parents, sisters, and other members of their primary support system have been unable to travel to be with them when they come home as new moms. The lack of physical and emotional support during the pandemic caused even more new parents to struggle with PMHDs. According to a 2022 brief from the World Health Organization, rates of anxiety and depression have increased by 25 percent in the general population since the COVID-19 pandemic, disproportionately affecting young people and women.[4] Similarly, there also has been a drastic increase in the rates of PMHDs. Pre-pandemic, the prevalence of PMHDs was 15 to 20 percent; however, studies after the height of the COVID-19 pandemic show rates up to 34 percent. PMHDs are the most common complication in pregnancy and postpartum (defined as the first year after birth).[5] These mental health disorders are not isolated to the birth parent alone. Partners also have a one-in-ten risk of developing postpartum depression.

We're finally on the precipice of a new time when the stigma surrounding mental health is lessening and more people, including prominent celebrities such as Chrissy Teigen and Adele, are opening up about their own struggles with mental health disorders. Creating a culture in which women feel comfortable speaking up about their symptoms is crucial, as many new parents suffer in silence for fear of being judged as weak, incompetent, crazy, or—even worse—as unfit mothers. They're afraid of Child Protective Services being called if they admit they're suffering from symptoms of depression. This fear is especially pronounced in marginalized communities, where many new parents are afraid to even admit to symptoms of postpartum depression. Their fears are valid. In 2022, Child Welfare Services acknowledged racial disparities and released recommendations to address them.[6]

We also know that the screeners used today, mainly the EPDS and the PHQ-9, are not as sensitive among Black birthing people and other marginalized groups. Additional screens for anxiety, stress, and post-traumatic stress disorder, which may better pick up the symptoms in some populations, are being developed and studied; however, we aren't yet at the point at which any have been validated and routinely implemented. Between the fear of reporting symptoms, the lack of quality mental health care resources when symptoms are reported, and the decreased sensitivity of screeners, many people are slipping through the cracks. Studies have shown Black birthing people are twice as likely to develop a PMHDs and half as likely to get the needed help.[7]

From my personal experience as an obstetrician, training taught me to only look out for the rare cases of severely depressed birthing parents who had thoughts of harming themselves or their babies. So when I developed severe anxiety, panic disorder, and obsessive compulsive behaviors after my daughter was born, I had no clue that this wasn't just the hypervigilance of a new mom. I thought it was normal to be unable to fall asleep and to imagine every possible scenario in which my child may get hurt. I thought it would get better as my daughter got older, but when she started crawling and putting things in her mouth, I continually imagined that she would choke on something or poison herself. I almost gave in to the industry created just for people like me: professional baby proofers who, for thousands of dollars, baby proof your home so that every possible disaster scenario can be mitigated. I doubt this would have assuaged my anxiety, though, as my mind readily moved on to the next available doomsday scenario.

My friends teased me because now that I was a mom, I went to bed at 8:00 p.m. This was because I was so exhausted from constantly being on high alert that I couldn't function by evening. It eventually got to the point that I could no longer enjoy many of the activities I used to or normal moments with my daughter without preparing for what may happen, and my anxiety became compounded by depression. Ironically, it was living in the epicenter of the COVID pandemic that finally gave me the path to reclaim my sanity.

The stress of COVID accelerated the decline of my mental health. I became so rundown that I had no energy to get through the day. It took all of my energy to maintain the focus necessary to get through the workday. I began to worry that I was suffering from an autoimmune disease or cancer. I had reached a low point, and I was forced to start searching for answers. I gained insight into my disorders when I read the article, "Is Fear the Last Taboo of Motherhood?" by Susannah Cahalan, published in the *New York Times* in 2020,[8] and, subsequently, the book *Ordinary Insanity*,[9] which is the subject of the article. Some of the initial stories in the book seemed very extreme to me, but as I kept reading, more and more of the stories resonated with me. I was dumbstruck.

How could I, a board-certified OB/GYN, have spent two years suffering and found myself on the precipice of an emotional breakdown before I was able to diagnose my own severe anxiety and depression? I went online and administered the Edinburgh Postpartum Depression Scale, a screening tool used for determining women at high risk for depression, to myself. I scored in the range consistent with symptoms of severe depression.

When I went for my postpartum visits, my obstetrician had never asked me pointed questions regarding anxiety, depression, PTSD, or OCD. She was very compassionate, but the topic of perinatal mood and anxiety disorders never once entered the conversation during my prenatal or postpartum care. This is very common; postpartum depression—along with everything else related to the diagnosis and treatment of mental health—is only now gaining the attention it deserves.

We're still a long way from where we need to be to have the necessary conversations, to normalize and destigmatize the diagnosis and treatment of mental health conditions, and to improve access to basic mental health services.

How did I not recognize my own diagnosis? OB/GYNs aren't trained to appropriately diagnose and treat these disorders. Only recently have providers started screening patients at their six-week postpartum visits for postpartum depression. However, the most common tools, the PHQ-9 and the EPDS, screen specifically for symptoms of depression, not anxiety, OCD, PTSD, or bipolar disorder.

In addition, women are often not asked how they're doing in a way that really identifies these symptoms. A lot of women say they're fine even when they're not, because they either think that what they're experiencing is normal or feel bad or guilty for not being a perfect mom. They believe they shouldn't have feelings other than the pure joy they believe they're "supposed" to feel after giving birth. I have had many friends tell me that they lied on the questionnaire so that they didn't "fail."

Many women, like me, also don't realize when their normal preoccupation with the baby tips over into clinical anxiety, panic disorder, or OCD. They may not be able to differentiate when their baby blues, which are almost universal, tip over into depression. Women also may have thoughts of harming themselves or their babies but won't admit to it unless asked targeted questions in a supportive environment where they feel safe. I have had conversations with women who are very placid and calm but admit to thoughts about killing themselves or drowning their baby when asked specific questions. For most, these are known as "intrusive thoughts." They're horrifying to the person experiencing them, who never wants to think about harming their baby, but they cannot keep the nightmarish images from popping into their head. Intrusive thoughts are extremely common, even in new parents without PMHDs.

For other new parents, thoughts of harming themselves or their baby are part of a belief that they need to find a way out and that killing themselves and/or their baby is the only way to escape the world they're living in. In postpartum psychosis, the thoughts also may be part of complex delusions or hallucinations in which they truly believe they must take their life and/or their baby's life. Postpartum psychosis is an emergency. If you think you or someone you love is experiencing symptoms of psychosis, please call 911 or go to your nearest hospital.

RISK FACTORS

Anyone can develop a perinatal mental health disorder, but there are certain risk factors you should be aware of. The most common risk factors for PMHDs are a personal history of anxiety, depression, or bipolar disorder (including a history of a PMHD), a family history of mental health conditions, or a history of sensitivity to hormonal shifts such as premenstrual dysphoric disorder. Knowing you're at risk and taking precautions even before you develop symptoms can help you avoid struggling during pregnancy and postpartum. Support groups, mindfulness practices, therapy, and medication are commonly utilized to help prevent and treat PMHDs. You can better prepare yourself with the best support and care to prevent PMHDs if you know you have risk factors for these disorders ahead of time.

PREVENTING AND TREATING PMHDS

If you suspect that you may be suffering with a PMHD, talk to your doctor right away. The following advice also can be helpful in preventing PMHDs or in healing emotionally as you seek professional support.

Sleep Is Medicine

In the immediate aftermath of having a baby, your body is pumped full of a lot of hormones, including cortisol, to help you focus on bonding with your baby and protecting and caring for your new infant. Cortisol may make you feel as if you don't need much sleep, and you may start to wonder what everyone was talking about. You feel great! Then the cortisol levels decrease, and you're left exhausted, depleted, and feeling helpless. You wonder if you'll ever get enough sleep to be a functioning human again. The good news is that this period does eventually end and you'll someday feel like a functioning human being again. Perhaps a very different human than you were pre-baby, but that's for another chapter.

One of my favorite people, Lisa Tremayne, a registered nurse and perinatal mental health specialist, is not only an expert in perinatal mental health, but also in sleep training. She started helping new parents get the support they need to increase their sleep because she knew this plays such a pivotal role in mental health. When I first met Lisa, she taught me something profound that has changed the way I counsel new parents about getting enough sleep: "Sleep is medicine," she said. "Think about what happens when someone has severe postpartum depression or psychosis and is admitted to the hospital. What do they do to treat them? They first take away all distractions and then give them enough sedatives so that they can sleep. This is so important to recovery."[10]

If you do not get enough sleep during the postpartum period, your body cannot recover from giving birth and your mind cannot function. Sleep deprivation can lead to irritability, communication issues with your partner, difficulty bonding with your baby, and, as it worsens, it can contribute significantly to the development of PMHDs. When I talk to a new parent who is hypervigilant and having such severe intrusive thoughts that they are not sleeping more than an hour or two at a stretch and cannot sleep when the baby is sleeping, the first thing I do is emphasize the importance of sleep and recommend something like a mild benzodiazepine to help her fall and stay asleep. Otherwise, I fear she may spiral into a dangerous place, which could include delusions, hallucinations, and mania, all of the really bad places the mind can go to when it is severely sleep deprived.

The goal, according to Lisa, is to get a minimum of six consecutive hours a night. This may sound like a fantasy during the postpartum period, but it is possible with the right support and prioritization. If you can't get it all overnight, nap when the baby is napping instead of trying to do other things around the home. Your sleep, your mental and emotional well-being, is more important for you and your baby than anything else on your to-do list. For new parents who are breastfeeding or chestfeeding around the clock in the early days, your partner or another support person can change the baby, bring the baby to you, burp the baby after the feed, and put the baby back to sleep. This will not eliminate sleep interruptions but it will minimize their duration. Other alternatives include pumping a supply of milk during the day and using pumped milk or formula overnight for at least one feed or fortifying some of your breast milk from the day with formula at night and having a support person do the nighttime feeds so you can sleep. While you are building your milk supply, breastfeeding or pumping every two to three hours is recommended to get the supply necessary to feed your baby exclusively via breast milk; however, once your supply is established, you can wean off of night feeds or pumping. The breasts function on supply and demand. If you space out the feeding frequency and duration at night, the breasts will accommodate this change in demand so that you are able to go longer overnight without becoming engorged, just as they do when the baby gets older and does not wake as frequently overnight to feed.

For many new parents, their infant feeding goal is exclusive breastfeeding. However, you should remember that the most important thing for your new baby is for you to be healthy. A parent who is not sleeping because they are awake and stressed about producing enough milk is going to suffer mentally, emotionally, and physically—and how you are feeling impacts your baby as well.

If you are unable to sleep when the baby is sleeping because you are having intrusive thoughts about something bad happening to the baby or if you have insomnia because you are stressing about everything that needs to be done around the house (or, worse, stay awake doing all of these things during the few critical hours you could be resting), this may be a sign of postpartum anxiety or postpartum obsessive compulsive disorder. Talk to your trusted healthcare provider if this is the case.

Treatment for PMHDs

There are many different pharmacologic and nonpharmacologic treatment options for perinatal mental health disorders. Depending on your diagnosis, symptoms, and the severity of your symptoms, different treatment options may be recommended. For more severe symptoms, a combination of therapy and antidepressant medication has been shown to resolve symptoms faster than using either alone. During the postpartum period, every day that you struggle with severe symptoms is a day that you cannot bond well with your baby. Additionally, you are at risk for worsening symptoms leading to the need for emergency treatment in the hospital, so time is of the essence. For milder symptoms, develop a personalized care plan with your provider. If your provider is not knowledgeable and comfortable counseling and speaking to you about the treatment options, please find someone who is.

There is so much shame and stigma surrounding mental health and taking antidepressants, especially during pregnancy and while breastfeeding. When I asked Dr. Lucy Hutner, a wonderful reproductive psychiatrist whom I have had the pleasure of collaborating with and learning from, how she addresses this when counseling her patients, she gave me this sage advice, which anyone who may be considering going on medication can use:

> Nothing we do in pregnancy and postpartum is solely about our heads; our hearts are involved too. Many patients feel tempted to do whatever they think will be "best" for the pregnancy and they feel like they should just "suck it up" and deal with poor mental health. I try to respect and honor their perspective while aiming to alleviate any guilt about getting the treatment they need. We have to learn to put our own oxygen masks on first—and that starts in pregnancy. Of course, stigma plays a role, too. Our society traditionally emphasizes an idea that you should just "get over" your depression or anxiety—which is then internalized by patients—rather than honoring it like any other medical condition. [The treatment plan] is a collaboration between decision-making partners—one person who has lived experience and will be going through it in real time, and the other with clinical expertise who can help to guide decision making.[11]

There are more and more perinatal mental health specialists in all aspects of mental health care, and I do recommend finding someone who has special training or who has developed this specific niche in their practice. Otherwise, they may not recognize the red flags that are common in postpartum depression and anxiety that are not outside of the peripartum period, or they might give inaccurate information and counseling regarding the safety of using antidepressants and other psychiatric medications during pregnancy and breastfeeding. I have had many patients with chronic underlying psychiatric diagnoses stop their medications when trying to conceive or upon finding out that they are pregnant because their provider recommended it. Please always get a consultation from a provider educated in medication management during pregnancy and breastfeeding, as there are often many risks associated with stopping your medication and potentially developing severe symptoms that outweigh the risks of staying on your medication. One of the best places to look for a list of specialists in your area is the Postpartum Support International (PSI) provider database. Providers like me who are passionate about caring for people with perinatal mental health disorders (and often have our own lived experiences that brought us to this work) are listed by state. You can also call the maternal mental health hotline, which is staffed by PSI counselors who can help you find resources that are available to you.

As for nonpharmacologic management, cognitive behavioral therapy is a cornerstone of treatment. Just as with medication, I recommend seeing a therapist with experience in caring for people who are pregnant and postpartum. The power of community also cannot be underestimated, and peer support groups are also really beneficial. Whether online or in person, talking to other new parents who can validate your feelings and experiences, especially those that do not line up with the glossy images we see and compare ourselves to, can be so helpful. Knowing that you are not alone, that everyone struggles, that everyone feels and does things on their parenting journey for which others may judge or criticize them, can be so reassuring and really help your mental and emotional state.

There are also many other complementary ways to boost your mental health, such as exercise, acupuncture, and ecotherapy (taking walks outside and looking at the flowers, listening to the birds, and getting some sunshine can ground and renew you). Dr. Anna Glezer,

MD, reproductive and integrative psychiatrist, routinely recommends magnesium supplements and high-dose omega-3 fish oils to her patients to help with the symptoms of anxiety and depression, as well as focusing on postpartum nutrition: protein sources for energy and anti-inflammatory foods are both important for healing and for mental health. Sometimes mental health symptoms can be attributed to or compounded by other underlying imbalances, so you can also ask your provider to check your blood count for anemia, your vitamin D levels, and your thyroid hormone, as conditions such as anemia and hypo- or hyperthyroid can lead to anxiety and mood symptoms. And, as Dr. Glezer counsels her patients and providers who enroll in her fellowship on integrative psychiatry, "Keep in mind there's also a difference between the normal blood levels and the optimal ones."[12] For example, in my practice most patients have vitamin D deficiency or are on the low end of the normal range (greater than 20 nanograms per milliliter is considered "normal"); however, to prevent and treat depression, I recommend my patients get their levels closer to 40 nanograms per milliliter. This usually requires taking a supplement.

BIRTH TRAUMA

According to the National Institutes of Health, the prevalence of individuals who report experiencing a traumatic birth event is up to 45 percent.[13] Although only a small percentage of people who experience birth trauma develop post-traumatic stress disorder, many birthing people who experience a traumatic event will exhibit some of the signs and symptoms of trauma, so it is very important to understand if you or a loved one may be experiencing birth trauma.

For this section, I spoke to some incredible perinatal trauma specialists. Much about this topic is best heard directly from the voices of those who have the professional skills to help others process their trauma. It is critical that those who experience symptoms of obstetric trauma find a professional to work through this with them when they are ready to process the experience. Trauma is insidious, and if it is not processed, it will continue to be triggered and affect your life in more ways than you may even recognize. It is important to process your trauma with a trauma specialist who is trained in special modalities of therapy that are trauma focused, such as eye movement desensitization and reprocessing (EMDR). It is also important to note that although you can talk about your experiences with your providers, family, and support system, having a professional who not only listens and holds space but understands how to respond when you are triggered as you unpack your trauma is really important for your emotional and mental recovery.

What Makes an Event Traumatic?

Dr. Jaz Robbins, psychologist and trauma specialist, advises that "it's important to recognize that 'birth trauma' is an umbrella term that encompasses many types of traumatic birthing experiences. These experiences can range from the birthing person being excluded from participating in important decisions, to them being physically harmed/assaulted, to complicated births that require emergency medical interventions. Birth trauma is a term that holds space for all of these experiences."[14]

Moreover, as all of the experts I spoke to reinforced, trauma is in the eye of the beholder. There is no formula for what makes an event traumatic. We all have unique lived experiences that have shaped our brains and our perceptions. As Julie Bindeman, reproductive psychologist, says, "It depends upon the individual nervous system and how it's going to respond to trauma being triggered."[15] This not only makes it hard to know what will be traumatic to someone, but it makes it difficult to prevent trauma on an individual level. We also do not know what will trigger someone with a history of trauma, so if you have trauma in your past, it is especially important to work with a specialist prior to giving birth so that you are better prepared with the right tools to help prevent and work through triggers that may happen during the birth process.

I have been present at many births that seemed to me to be beautiful experiences without any untoward interventions or complications; however, when I spoke to the birth person postpartum, they told me it was awful because they felt so out of control of their own body during the experience. I have also had patients who had emergency

C-sections or massive hemorrhages and I was very worried about how they would process the experience—but they told me that they felt like everything was explained to them thoroughly, all of their questions were answered, and they trusted the team taking care of them. They overall felt that their birth experience was a positive one and were grateful that they and their baby are healthy.

How Does Trauma Look?

According to Dr. Bindeman, trauma can look very different for different people, so it may be hard to recognize, but there are some signs to look for. She recommends being aware of how the birthing person interacts with the baby: "One of the hardest things in a birth trauma is that the baby was the source of the trauma, or at least was part of the circumstance of that trauma. And then you have this constant exposure and you are supposed to interact a certain way with the very being that traumatized you."

Other signs include dissociating, spacing out, or being unable to track conversation, being prone to anger, lashing out, or defensiveness, acting really withdrawn or quiet, or being nervous about other people being near the baby. Dr. Bindeman also notes that some of these symptoms can overlap with other perinatal mental health disorders, and often it requires a professional to get the right diagnosis.

How Does Trauma Feel?

Dr. Kelsey Power, another perinatal trauma specialist, has heard her clients describe their trauma in many different ways. Examples she gave me include:

- Disconnection: You might feel like you're not present in moment-to-moment experiences.
- Guilt and shame: Is there a voice that has become more active in terms of how you think about yourself?
- Intrusive thoughts: Disturbing thoughts come into your head that you can't control.

- Alienation: You may be isolating yourself or feeling like you don't want to see anyone.
- Disassociation: Do you recognize yourself? Are there aspects of your experience of yourself that feel foreign or unreal?
- Distrust: Do you find that you are becoming less trusting of people around you or that people are judging you?
- Insecurity: You feel like environments or relationships that once felt secure no longer feel so friendly or so supportive.[16]

Do Not Compare Your Trauma to Others

It is important not to minimize your own experience by comparing your trauma to that of others. Your trauma deserves attention and care. Just because you did not experience a catastrophic event such as a near-death experience does not mean you should dismiss your own experience. If it is affecting you, tell others and get the help and support you deserve. Your loved ones can help by setting up an appointment for you and even taking you to your appointment. They can also help by keeping aspects of your routine and day predictable. You may not know what will trigger your trauma, so having trusted people surrounding and supporting you and maintaining a set flow to your days can help minimize unanticipated events that may lead to trauma being triggered. Structure and a sense of safety and security in your environment, especially the sensory inputs and the people that are around you, can be helpful.

Secondary Trauma

It is also very important to recognize that anyone who was present when the trauma occurred may experience secondary trauma. Your loved one may have witnessed you go through an experience that was really scary, when they felt like you or the baby were not safe or were suffering and were not being cared for properly. They often feel helpless and out of control in these situations and also can experience trauma from these events. If you are a loved one who witnessed a traumatic event, make sure that you also get the support you need to process your secondary trauma.

ADDITIONAL RESOURCES FOR TRAUMA AND PMHDS

There are many online resources, support groups, and hotlines to help women who are suffering from any of the disorders along the spectrum of peripartum mood and anxiety disorders and those who have risk factors for PMHDs. Be proactive in getting support and care to prevent symptoms from even developing. The largest online resource is Postpartum Support International (PSI), which offers a wealth of helpful resources on its website, including access to a warm call line to help you find professional support in your area and free weekly support groups. In 2022, Health Resources and Services Administration (HRSA) launched a national 24/7 warm call line staffed by experts from PSI.

For emergencies, including thoughts of harming yourself or your baby, please put your baby in a safe place such as a crib and call or text 988, the National Suicide and Crisis hotline, to reach someone 24/7. For nonemergency support, call 1-833-TLC-MAMA, the 24/7 warm line set up through HRSA and staffed by counselors who can help you when you really need to connect with someone for support and validation.

WORDS OF SUPPORT

We all need to become more comfortable having conversations regarding mental health, especially when it affects new parents and their babies during such a vulnerable and critical time in their lives. All new parents should feel empowered to speak up for themselves and ask for help without fear of judgment. Do it for yourself, your baby, and your family. If you think you may be suffering from a perinatal mood or anxiety disorder, always ask for help from your doctor, midwife, nurse, family, friends, or by accessing the resources mentioned earlier.

If someone you care about is pregnant or has recently given birth, ask them specific questions about how they're feeling and really listen to their responses. Also take the time to ask the partners how they're coping, as either or both partners may have postpartum depression. It is very stressful, making it very difficult to function and cope.

Please share my words of support and education for new parents in your life who may be struggling with PMHDs:

- PMHDs are pervasive. They may affect parents of any background, even if they don't have risk factors, even if this is not their first baby and they never developed symptoms before.
- You're not a bad parent or a weak person. We are all human and we all have struggles.
- Don't try to "tough it out." Without proper care and support, symptoms typically persist and may progressively worsen.
- These conditions are treatable! With the right treatment, you will get better.

My own experience with postpartum anxiety, depression, and OCD was a long journey since it took me so long to recognize the conditions in myself. However, once I treated it, I started to feel better almost immediately. For me, the first step was starting antidepressants. From there, I was able to release some of the anxious thoughts and guilt regarding not doing everything myself, which in turn led me to set boundaries and ask for help, ultimately giving me the mental bandwidth to take time for therapy and other forms of self-care. During my second pregnancy, I was on antidepressants and in therapy the whole time and I had a much better postpartum experience, the type of experience that I hope that all of you can have as well with the right tools and support in place.

TEN

FEEDING YOUR BABY

In the 1990s, the World Health Organization (WHO) and UNICEF launched the Baby-Friendly Hospital Initiative to encourage health-care providers to offer more support for new birthing parents and to promote breastfeeding. The campaign was best known for its now-infamous motto: "Breast is best." The campaign was hugely successful and created intense societal pressure among birthing people to exclusively breastfeed.

Despite good intentions, the campaign was mostly misguided and failed to take into account how many new parents struggle with breastfeeding/chestfeeding. Lack of supply, problems latching, painful, cracked, or bleeding nipples, mastitis (infection in the breast), or a combination of these can lead to what has been called in recent studies a "lactastrophe." Moreover, breastfeeding is an intensely personal and intimate experience, filled with the complex interplay of hormones, your unique body, and your unique baby. We also live in a society that does not support breastfeeding and new parenthood in general. With very little paid maternity/paternity leave and often inadequate time or space at work to pump, even those who exclusively breastfeed before returning to work either end up with decreased supply or just quit because it is too much of a struggle to maintain a regular pumping routine. It's too simplistic to say "breast is best" and assume that guidance will work for everyone.

WHY THE FOCUS ON BREASTFEEDING?

The mantra "breast is best" is reinforced in the structures of our healthcare system and in society. Hospitals pay to be accredited by Baby-Friendly USA, and one of the major standards for the Baby-Friendly Hospital designation is that they must encourage and report their rates of exclusive breastfeeding upon discharge. In addition, the Baby-Friendly Hospital Initiative Interim Guidelines, updated November 2019, states, "Step 6: Give infants no food or drink other than breast milk, unless medically indicated. Exclusive breast milk feeding shall be the feeding method expected from birth to discharge. Each facility should track its rate of formula supplementation of breastfed infants. Facilities should strive to reach the Healthy People 2020 goal for exclusive breastfeeding."[1]

Although exclusive breastfeeding on discharge has become the gold standard for hospitals, this goal is unrealistic. Up to 15 percent of birthing people will never be able to exclusively breastfeed, and those who eventually do often require supplementation while establishing their milk supply. The US Department of Health and Human Services Healthy People 2020 guidelines set a target of only 14.2 percent of infants receiving any formula supplementation during the first two days of life.[2]

Most of my patients and friends have wanted to exclusively breastfeed their babies. I did as well. I wanted to make sure my baby received my antibodies, because I happen to have an amazing immune system due to growing up with two parents who worked in the hospital and a family dog (yes, dogs do help your immune system!). I also wanted to check the box that made me feel like a good mom and gave my child the best chance of getting into the university of her choice and succeeding in life. Because if breast is best, why would I ever feed my child anything else? That would automatically categorize me as a "bad mom."

According to Christie del Castillo-Hegyi, an emergency physician and cofounder of the Fed Is Best Foundation, "One of the biggest dangers of the Breast is Best initiative, and the WHO guidelines to exclusively breastfeed for the first six months of an infant's life, is that while they recommend exclusive breastfeeding for the first six months of life, they do not acknowledge that for many new parents, exclusive breastfeeding is not even physiologically possible."[3] Marianne Neifert, MD, the cofounder of the Academy of Breastfeeding

Medicine, studied healthy women with full-term babies who were motivated to exclusively breastfeed. Even with extensive support to achieve this goal (which most new parents do not have), 15 percent, or one in seven, had persistent low milk supply. And we don't even know what the rates of low supply are beyond one month.[4]

"It's such an unfair standard," says Dr. del Castillo-Hegyi. "It's just a cruel lie to tell people that you will succeed if you follow XYZ, and if you don't succeed, you did something wrong. You weren't educated or you didn't try hard enough. It's the worst possible message a postpartum mom could possibly receive. It's so heartbreaking, and you don't understand it until you've gone through it. I had denial [that I couldn't exclusively breastfeed]. You're so anxious about things going right that you kind of block out anyone who says, 'Well, sometimes it doesn't go that way.' You just have to be prepared."

Breastfeeding is the most natural way to feed our babies. It can be a bonding experience with our babies. It has purported health benefits. But should the gold standard be an exclusively breastfed baby, or should it be a thriving, well-fed baby? Often these two objectives conflict, leaving many new parents struggling to maintain the standard set by the WHO and society and also to ensure their babies are not failing to thrive. Due to the recent formula shortage and the shaming of moms who are formula feeding that ensued, Emily Oster released for free the full chapter "Breast Is Best? Breast Is Better? Breast Is about the Same?" from her book *Cribsheets*. This is an excellent resource that delves further into the data available on the benefits of breastfeeding and demonstrates that a majority of the claims don't have substantial high-quality data to back them up. According to Dr. Oster, for full-term and near-term babies, "it seems reasonable to conclude that breastfeeding lowers infant eczema and gastrointestinal infections. For the other illness outcomes, the most compelling evidence is in favor of a small reduction in ear infections in breastfed children."[5] It is important to note that the data is based on studies done in countries like the United States, where there is clean drinking water and good quality formula available.

Breastfeeding can be a beautiful bonding opportunity and an empowering experience for some people, but others may find that it affects them negatively both physically and mentally. Struggles with breastfeeding are one of the most common risk factors for postpartum anxiety and depression, not in small part due to the connection with sleep deprivation and the stress related to continual worry about whether your baby is getting enough food. Besides the lack of data showing any long-term health or cognitive benefits and the minimal short-term health benefits among full-term infants, there are also many challenges and complications that new parents face when breastfeeding and pumping, which can make the experience unpleasant at best and something they dread at worst.

THE CHALLENGES OF BREASTFEEDING

Many expecting parents envision that because breastfeeding is natural, it will be easy. They're then surprised, disappointed, or feel like failures when they struggle. Concern about low supply is also a common stressor for many new parents, and struggles with breastfeeding are one of the most common factors leading to sleep deprivation and the development of perinatal mood and anxiety disorders. There is also often not enough support and education both in the hospital and after discharge. When new parents return to work—which, in the United States, with its lack of maternity leave support, is often much earlier than in other developed countries—the rates of exclusive breastfeeding drops even more. Although most infants born in 2017 started breastfeeding (84.1%), only 58.3 percent of infants were still breastfeeding at six months.[6]

Difficulties with breastfeeding/chestfeeding include the following.

Sore Nipples

Especially when initiating breastfeeding/chestfeeding, nipples will become sore, even if the baby has a good latch and is feeding well. There can be cracking, bleeding, and pain as well. Our nipples aren't used to the constant pulling and sucking of a new infant, and they must "toughen up," just like your hands would when playing a string instrument or doing manual work for the first time. Icing the nipples prior to latching and using nipple ointments after feeding can help create a barrier. Sometimes, if the pain is bad, giving your breasts some rest by taking a break and pumping on a lower setting for a few days can help.

Engorged Breasts

When milk comes in for the first time, new moms are often surprised by how uncomfortable and painful engorgement can be. This can happen at other times when the supply is greater than the demand or when a mom is away from her baby or in a place where she cannot take a break to breastfeed or pump. Often new moms are concerned that engorged breasts are a sign of mastitis, because engorgement can be painful and the breasts are hard, swollen, and warm to the touch. After breastfeeding or pumping, cold compresses can be applied and ibuprofen can be taken to decrease inflammation. Over time, supply and demand tend to even out, so unless you miss a feeding, engorgement shouldn't be as severe.

Mastitis

Mastitis is a condition in which an area of the breast has a clogged duct that cannot be released, leading to pain, redness, and fever. If you experience this, reach out to your provider. Occasionally antibiotics are warranted; however, most of the time mastitis is a sign of inflammation and not underlying infection. Cold compresses or ice packs also can help with the inflammation and blockage that causes mastitis. Massage is no longer recommended, because that can lead to further inflammation in the tissue. The recommended first-line antibiotics prescribed are safe during breastfeeding. Mastitis is not a medical reason to stop breastfeeding; continued breastfeeding or pumping actually can help the infection resolve. Rarely, the mastitis doesn't resolve with antibiotics, so if symptoms continue to worsen, reach out to your provider again, because an abscess may have developed. This is a walled-off collection of infection that's a rare but serious complication. It may need to be surgically drained to resolve.

Leaking Milk

This is extremely common, especially with engorgement, nipple stimulation, or hearing your baby cry. It is not dangerous, but it can be annoying or embarrassing. Nipple pads can be worn in your bra or shirt, and if the nipples are raw or sore, a small amount of ointment can be applied where these pads touch your sensitive nipples. This may help create an additional barrier between leaking milk and wet spots on your shirt.

Painful Latch

A painful latch can be a sign that the baby is not latching well. However, it also can be a sign of infection or cracked nipples. Painful latches should be evaluated by a certified lactation consultant or another healthcare provider to determine the cause. Sometimes it simply requires further education about how to latch the baby. Other times, it may require more help, such as nipple shields or even the release of a tongue or lip tie for the baby. If there is evidence of infection or cracked nipples, your obstetric provider can prescribe appropriate antibiotics or recommendations as noted earlier for sore nipples.

Failure to Latch

Failure to latch may be related to multiple factors from the shape of the nipple and breast to a baby with a tongue or lip tie. These physiologic variants aren't your fault and sometimes just take time and practice to make it work. Sometimes, however, it requires a professional to assess and make recommendations. If you're concerned that the baby is not latching or feeding well, call a lactation consultant or your pediatric provider. Until you figure out the cause and solution, you can pump and bottle feed or supplement with formula as necessary. If your baby previously was latching fine and then stops and seems disinterested in eating or is lethargic, call your pediatrician immediately.

Dysphoric Milk Ejection Reflex (DMER)

DMER is a medical condition caused by a drop in the hormone dopamine when oxytocin is released with milk letdown.[7] This occurs in a small percentage of breastfeeding/chestfeeding and pumping individuals and can lead to dysphoria, self-loathing, and other negative feelings that last for a few minutes at most. Others describe the sensation as a pit in their stomach. This can lead new parents to dread milk letdown and to feel alone, as it is a condition that is not often discussed. Many clinicians are not even aware of it, and there are no definitive treatments. However, for those suffering with it, often just knowing it has a name and that they are not alone helps.

LOW SUPPLY—IS MY BABY GETTING ENOUGH MILK?

With breastfeeding/chestfeeding, the amount of milk the baby is getting per breast, per feeding is not known, which leads many new parents to worry about whether the baby is getting enough milk. Your pediatrician will give you guidelines for the number of wet and soiled diapers to expect. They'll also be monitoring the baby's weight closely during the first few weeks, and longer if necessary, to make sure the baby regains the weight lost after birth and continues to thrive. They'll let you know if there are any concerning signs or symptoms and when supplementation is medically necessary. Lactation consultants and your pediatric team can work with you to develop a good feeding plan that ensures both you and your baby are healthy and thriving.

Dr. del Castillo-Hegyi has heard countless stories from parents whose children were diagnosed with failure to thrive, even though the moms had been working day and night for weeks to exclusively breastfeed. When the pediatrician tells them the baby is starving and they give the first formula bottle, the moms describe "feeling that not only did I fail, my breasts failed, my body failed, but I made my child go through weeks of hunger all because I was told that if your body doesn't produce enough, then you are doing it wrong or you just didn't get the right help or you're a rare biological anomaly." This is heartbreaking and a failure of providers and health organizations to

EARLY SIGNS THAT YOUR BABY IS UNDERFED AND REQUIRES SUPPLEMENTATION

- Feeding more frequently than every two hours all day long (different than cluster feeding, currently defined as two to three hours of more frequent feeding, which is fine)
- Crying all the time
- Frequent latching and unlatching

Late Signs of Starvation/Severe Dehydration*
- Hypoglycemia
- Jaundice
- Seizures
- The baby looks physically ill

*Some of these late signs are signs that brain injury has already occurred—you want to avoid getting to this point.

appropriately counsel new parents about the fact that some people simply will not produce enough milk to exclusively breastfeed.

Dr. del Castillo-Hegyi recommends new parents use an online newborn weight tool (https://newbornweight.org/), which allows you to track your child's weight during the first days and weeks compared to a large sample of children, which can help with earlier identification of weight loss and gain issues.[8]

I can't discuss low milk supply without mentioning triple feeding. Triple feeding is a method often recommended by lactation consultants and other professionals to help new parents increase their breast milk supply. This involves breastfeeding the baby, pumping, and giving the baby a formula bottle to supplement during the same feeding session. If a baby is feeding every two to three hours, you can imagine that between these three steps there is very little time for the new parent to do anything else other than work on increasing her milk supply and feeding the baby. I have seen moms completely miserable, exhausted from sleep deprivation and suffering with severe anxiety and depression. Triple feeding is meant to be for a very short time—just four to seven days, according to Dr. del Castillo-Hegyi. If your supply is not increasing at that point, it's probably not going to increase. Triple feeds is not meant to be a long-term feeding method. I have met new parents at their postpartum visits who have been trying to do triple feeds for weeks to months and were still under the impression their supply may increase if they just keep doing the work, even if it means losing their sanity and having no time to bond with their baby because they are pursuing exclusive breastfeeding.

If you are using formula or pumping and bottle feeding, here are some pro tips from lactation consultant Lynnette Hafken, a lactation and infant feeding consultant:

> One of the biggest misconceptions is that some baby formulas are higher quality, or more like breast milk, than others; there is a lot of marketing to convince parents that one formula is better than another, but in reality, all standard formulas are nutritionally equivalent. The same is true with bottles and nipples—we have theories, but no factual evidence to be able to say a certain shape, size, firmness, or flow rate is the best for all breastfed babies. Each human nipple varies in many ways, and breasts flow faster or slower depending on many factors (one side may have a fire hose letdown and the other a more gentle trickle). For all the baby knows, the bottle is mom's third breast, and they will adjust to it like they've adjusted to their mother's real nipples and milk flow. Babies are smarter than we sometimes give them credit for, and research is increasingly showing how flexible they can be.[9]

MY BREASTFEEDING EXPERIENCE

My personal experience with breastfeeding has made me a more empathetic person, and I'm now better able to counsel my patients and discuss this topic that new parents tend to have very strong feelings about. I personally didn't have a radiant glow around me during my days of lactation nor did I feel the intense bonding that many women report when either of my daughters latched on. I felt more like a dairy cow whose body is no longer their own and whose daily routine revolves around the cycle of producing milk, relinquishing that milk, and then consuming calories to produce more milk.

Everyone's experience and emotions regarding breastfeeding are different, and I assure you that if you're able to have a candid conversation with the people in your life whom you trust, you'll hear a wide variety of breastfeeding/chestfeeding stories and struggles. Here is a recap of my experience with breastfeeding.

I had a cesarean birth right before midnight but made sure that bright and early the next morning, while sleep deprived, still in shock, and my incision feeling like a hot knife was cutting into me, I slowly made my way down the hospital corridor to meet with the lactation consultant. I wasn't going to miss the group breastfeeding class, because that would mean I was already failing at being the best mom possible.

Six brand-new moms who had never met each other sat in a circle with the lactation consultant, whom we'd also never met. She introduced herself and immediately encouraged us all to drop our shirts so she could examine our nipples and squeeze them to see if colostrum came out. She cheered for those who easily expressed colostrum and demonstrated colostrum release on their breasts to the class. She reassured those whose bodies weren't as successful at on-demand performance. She then taught us the different positions for holding the baby while breastfeeding and helped us latch our babies.

That day, I lost any remaining modesty I had briefly held on to after my birth experience. It was in this class that I realized I'd never again have the same level of bodily privacy or autonomy I had maintained for my entire adult life. But this seemed normal and rational. Being selfless is part of the societal definition of being a good mom. It is only natural that you should embrace exposing your breasts to a room full of strangers in the pursuit of breastfeeding.

I can only imagine how this experience must feel for women who aren't professionals who spend their days giving other women breast exams, as well as women from more conservative cultures and those with a history of trauma, abuse, body shame, or gender dysphoria. Perhaps breastfeeding is empowering to them. Perhaps they're as bewildered by this experience as I was. Perhaps they're triggered from past trauma and experiences of loss of their bodily autonomy. Perhaps they're able to reclaim and re-identify with their body in a new way through the act of feeding their baby.

Postpartum day two, I experienced milk letdown. I really don't have adequate words to fully describe how this felt, but I'll try my best. I looked in the mirror at my huge, rock-hard, painful breasts and felt like a porn star from the 1980s with a bad boob job. Where had my body gone? Added to the fresh, red, swollen, and bruised 12-centimeter scar on my abdomen, the puffy, edematous body, and the dark circles under my eyes, I now also had a new pair of breasts that didn't resemble my own in the least. It was such a disorienting experience. All the nurses encouraged me that it was great my milk had come in so quickly! Some women wait anxiously for five days for their letdown. There was no room for thinking about my rapidly changing physicality in this world of being a new mom. I should feel only grateful for the abundance of milk I was gifted; feeling anything else would be narcissistic.

When I was discharged from the hospital, I had a nanny at home to help me while I recovered—a stranger whom I had never met, in my home, watching me as I struggled to walk around, fresh from major surgery, with my robe agape and my huge, painful, leaking breasts on display. Still, she was lovely and enthusiastic, informing me that it was best to breastfeed and then pump immediately afterward to increase my milk supply. This completely destroyed and remade my nipples. Those soft, sensitive structures packed with nerve endings experienced sharp pains, chafing, cracking, and bleeding during the first few weeks until they "toughened up." (Yes, this is a real thing. All moms who've breastfed can tell you your nipples are never the same after.) I also mastered a meticulous routine with nipple creams and figured out the proper settings and flange size on my breast pump. I was an enthusiastic student eager to do everything right and continued breastfeeding and pumping even as my body tried to tell me to slow down.

Breasts work on a supply-and-demand model in conjunction with our individual, naturally predetermined maximum milk production and storage capacities. Combined, these variants determine how much milk each woman can produce under optimal circumstances. I unknowingly had a family history of being "overproducers." I rapidly began producing more milk than one baby could ever need. My daughter couldn't even latch and properly feed, as she was choking on the forceful milk being expelled by my breasts. She was frustrated, I was frustrated, and my breasts were just angry.

For the rest of the moms out there, if you aren't producing a lot of milk, you may be genetically predisposed to produce less milk or have less capacity to store it. Two studies found that breast storage capacity can vary substantially between 2.6 and 20.5 ounces. This means that moms on the lower end of storage capacity could accumulate only 20 percent of the baby's milk intake at a time, whereas moms with the largest capacity could store up to 90 percent of the baby's daily milk intake at one time![10] Please don't blame yourself or feel like a failure if, after trying everything, you're still not producing enough to exclusively breastfeed, because it may be related to your anatomy.

For evidence-based resources and guidance, please see the resources at the end of the book. You can also ask your hospital, obstetric provider, or pediatrician for local trusted resources and certified lactation consultants who will work with you to achieve your goals but who will also honestly let you know when supplementation is recommended and safest for you or your baby's health.

Sometimes the stress and pressure to produce enough milk and exclusively breastfeed actually leads to decreased milk production. Sometimes if you have had a prolonged, intense labor and delivery, your baby went to the NICU, or you had a hemorrhage, your milk supply may decrease in the short term. In any case, supplementing a little with formula or donor milk decreases the pressure on you to perform, and the lower stress helps to improve your production. This doesn't mean you can't go back to exclusively breastfeeding when your supply increases, but if your baby is losing weight or not gaining weight, not peeing, or becoming jaundiced, then you need to seek medical advice and supplement when recommended by your provider.

I eventually learned a routine that worked best for me: pumping and bottle feeding the breast milk, then freezing the extra. Throughout my maternity leave, I pumped and stored a whole deep freezer full of milk that was eventually thrown away with many tears and curses when I realized my daughter would not drink it due to the high levels of lipase activity in my pumped milk (something else I had never been warned about that some people experience—it gives the milk a soapy smell and taste, which causes some babies to reject it, although other babies do not mind the taste). The lipase activity can be minimized by immediately heating and then freezing the milk after it is pumped—if you have the abundant time and desire to undertake such a task.

Throughout my first maternity leave, I continued to arrange my daily schedule and activities exclusively around my dates with the breast pump. I also experienced an airport that didn't have pumping rooms or an outlet in the bathroom, so my milk literally backed up into my armpits and I was crying in pain by the time I reached a safe, clean place to pump.

When I returned to work, I came back to an employer that didn't give me pump breaks or a relaxing place to pump during the few minutes I could steal away between patients. I quickly cut back and then stopped pumping during the day so my daughter would get breast milk in the morning and evening. By this time, with the help of birth control pills and decreased demand, my production slowed enough that she could tolerate latching. She eventually stopped wanting to latch at eight months. I was fine with this. I didn't mourn the loss of the baby-to-breast experience and was quite happy supplementing her diet with formula.

This was my experience. I should feel lucky. I produced enough milk to exclusively breastfeed my child for her first three months. She didn't have colic, allergies, elevated bilirubin, or weight loss. We didn't require intervention from the pediatrician, a lactation consultant, a tongue or lip tie released, or experience the exhausting trial and error of finding the perfect formula that a very sensitive or small baby requires.

Many parents would have traded anything to have my milk supply. I speak to women every day who are on the verge of an emotional breakdown, feeling exhausted and like a failure as a mom and woman because they have low milk production, problems latching, or both.

They devote their entire day and night to trying to stimulate the production breast milk for their babies. They use the nipple shields, massage their breasts with Epsom salts, and try every sort of supplement (teas, pills, powders, and even cookies) marketed as having properties to increase milk supply. I have seen countless women with postpartum depression due to their struggles with breastfeeding and the lack of sleep that ensues. I try to talk them off the ledge with some of the sentiments below.

Please share my words or your own encouraging variation with friends and family members who may need permission to stop their downward spiral of shame and guilt.

- Sleep deprivation, stress, guilt, depression, and anxiety aren't good for your baby. Your mission to exclusively breastfeed or to continue breastfeeding may be causing more harm than good for both of you.
- You're still an amazing parent if you supplement or stop breastfeeding. Treat yourself with compassion and stop judging yourself or worrying about others judging you.
- Give yourself permission to not force breastfeeding if it's not working for you or you just don't like it. Moms aren't meant to be martyrs. Having a happy, thriving parent is the most important gift you can give to your baby.

I don't deny that breastfeeding may be a beautiful and natural bonding experience that has numerous benefits for your growing baby. I'm in awe of every new parent who does it so easily and without complaint. But it's not for all of us. Did I try it again after my second child was born? I did; however, not for as long as the first time, and I made sure in advance to sign up to donate the excess to my local milk bank. Is it selfish to formula feed? Not from my point of view.

Sometimes not breastfeeding is a much-needed form of self-care. Sometimes breastfeeding is not possible due to medications the mom needs to take for her own health or for anatomical reasons. Sometimes breastfeeding triggers past traumas such as sexual abuse. I always ask patients how feeding is going during their postpartum visit and discuss any questions or concerns that they may have. Often if a new parent is not breastfeeding or is supplementing, they will apologetically or guiltily report this and feel the need to explain why.

Once I had a mom tell me, "I graduated from breastfeeding." She said this with a smile on her face. No guilt, shame, or justification offered. This mom was happy and thriving. She did what was right for her and her baby, no matter the reason, and without fear of judgment. I loved her attitude, the self-compassion she displayed with that simple response. No matter what your feeding journey entails, I hope that you treat yourself with the same self-compassion and that you also treat other moms—whether breastfeeding or bottle feeding, topless in the park or pumping in a bathroom—without judgment and with the same compassionate support that we all deserve.

When creating your own feeding plan, keep in mind your overarching goals as a new parent. "Think about what you want for your baby, and then think about what you want for yourself, and then think about what you want for what your family looks like. The idea of saying that you're important and that your sleep is important, your mental health is important, is a radical thought to some women," reflects Dr. del Castillo-Hegyi.

I strongly agree with this perspective and often advocate for my patients to consider all aspects of how exclusively breastfeeding (or breastfeeding/pumping in any amount) impacts their health and well-being as well as that of their baby. If breastfeeding is something that you enjoy, great. If not, think about the real reasons why you are forcing yourself to struggle through the experience. Breastfeeding is not synonymous with being a good mom, and not breastfeeding is not synonymous with being a bad mom. If you are breastfeeding or pumping because it's how you "should" feed your baby, and self-sacrifice is what mothers "should" embody, then I want to give you permission to stop and choose a feeding method that meets the needs of you and your family.

For all of you who are on or will be on this messy, imperfect journey and still struggle to find out what makes sense for you and your family, I end this chapter with the beautiful wisdom from Lynnette Hafken (I cried the first time I read it):

What is the baby experiencing during this process? Just how valuable is more breast milk compared with more snuggles? If these seem like impossible questions, they often are, because we do not have the ingredients to raising a child perfectly. We raise them like humans, imperfect, and hopefully accepting that we're good enough for them as we are. We *are* good enough—children don't want perfection, they want *us*, their own parents. Accepting yourself as you are—teaching your child compassion and forgiveness over self-criticism—is the real "best."

ELEVEN

EXERCISE AND NUTRITION AFTER BABY

Exercise after birth is another area that caught me by surprise as a new mom. I worked out regularly up until the end of my pregnancy, having no idea just how weak I'd be after delivery. I didn't know which exercises were safe or not safe. I also had to learn how to stop the self-criticism and treat my body with grace—after all, I had just grown and birthed a human being. Many birthing people are so sleep deprived and sore from carrying around a baby that doing anything other than pushing the stroller may seem unattainable at first. This is okay! Everyone must resume their normal activities at their own pace and should never feel bad that they don't look like the models or yoga instructors on Instagram by six weeks postpartum. This chapter helps you learn how to safely start working out again and what new sensations to expect.

After my first daughter was born, I looked in the mirror and did not recognize myself. It was extremely disorienting. Based on what society had taught me, I should look and feel like nothing had happened. Instead, I felt like my body was a broken version of what it had previously been. I felt the intense pressure to "bounce back," to look as if nothing had happened, as if I had not just birthed a human into the world and undergone major abdominal surgery. If I had a more realistic expectation of what to anticipate, I would have more readily accepted and formed a healthier relationship with my new body. I hope that this chapter helps you understand some of the changes your body undergoes and how that impacts your fitness postpartum, as well as how to approach exercise when you feel ready to get back to it.

I also provide basic nutritional advice in this chapter. Although your focus may be ensuring that your baby is getting enough food, you also need to be nourished properly to recover from giving birth and to produce food for your baby, if you are breastfeeding/chestfeeding.

RECOVER FIRST

Before stepping right back into exercise and resuming your pre-pregnancy or pre-baby activities, realize that you'll need to spend some time in recovery. This can be hard for a lot of patients, and many birthing people try to cut short their recovery before they're truly ready.

Ronit Sukenick, an amazing pelvic floor physical therapist, has worked with people before and after giving birth for many years. She also has her own lived experience with a long postpartum recovery that gives her additional insight and empathy when working with her clients. She suggested another way to look at the downtime before you are cleared to really work on your corrective exercises and active recovery. "Relish and enjoy that there's actually a recovery time," says Ronit.

> When you are doing basic things that you did when you were pregnant, notice how they are different now. And appreciate doing the things you couldn't do before because you were pregnant. There's actually a recovery that has to happen. It's not just tissue recovery that has to happen. There's things that actually have to happen to recover and get better and you have to respect those things. [In the meantime,] you can walk as much as you want. You're not trying to beat your personal record here; you're just walking for enjoyment to get out in the sun, getting some fresh air. Look at how you're doing things now that you're not pregnant anymore. If you're doing things that still are the things you did when you were pregnant, like walking in a waddle, you can start to think about how you don't need to waddle anymore. Or [recognizing that] you don't have that same situation anymore, like getting out of bed in a very specific way or lifting your hips when you move in bed instead of rolling. You can roll now. You're going to feel much freer. Look at what you're doing and kind of be like, "Oh, I don't have to do it that way anymore." Like lying on your belly, which you haven't done in so long, or do

some cobras and just open up again. Do the things you haven't done in so long because they're going to all feel ridiculously hard or stiff or weird. The whole point of rehabbing you is getting you back to how you moved before.[1]

Ronit's words remind us that there's a period of time when we should gently get to know our new bodies and learn how they work again. At the same time, you might enjoy the simple pleasures of movement unencumbered by a large pregnant belly before thinking about getting back to exercising.

DON'T EXPECT TO "BOUNCE BACK"

There are many images that can be harmful for a newly postpartum person to see, especially the ones on social media showing how someone "bounced back" just weeks after their delivery. I applaud people for feeling empowered and proud of their bodies after having a baby. I wish everyone did, no matter what their bodies look like and how long it takes them to get back to a physical place where they feel comfortable in their own skin. Growing and birthing a human, as you know now, is a physically intense experience. No two healing journeys are the same, and if you have had more than one birth experience, each post-birth recovery will be different.

No matter how you feel about your body after giving birth, the goal of "bouncing back" is unrealistic. There are some people who exercise their whole pregnancy, are thin, young, gain little weight throughout the pregnancy, and have a smooth birth experience who may appear to quickly return to a physically similar state to what they were prepregnancy, with or without exercise. However, physical appearance is only a small part of it. Alignment, strength, and stamina are also impacted by pregnancy. Exercising too soon and progressing too quickly after birth can be harmful to your body, no matter what it looks like.

Joanie Johnson, a wonderful perinatal trainer who works in person with clients as well as through her web-based subscription platform *Transformation Nation*, helped me a lot through her online platform after my first daughter was born. Joanie, like me, has the lived experience of being surprised by the slow pace of her post-birth recovery. Joanie is not only a trainer but also had been a professional dancer for many years prior to her pregnancy and cesarean birth. As Joanie told me, "Some people think a 'bounce back' is going to be easy, especially people who are extremely fit, myself as an example. I checked all of the boxes and I had a very long and hard recovery and it was really humbling. Your mental state is a big part of it."[2]

START SMALL

After the birth of my second daughter, I worked with perinatal trainer Brianna Houston to help me recover in a very conscious way. I knew that after my second C-section, there would be more scar tissue and nerve damage, so I would need to be very careful to heal and exercise appropriately. I learned so much about my body and how to reconnect to my core and pelvic floor that I otherwise never would have understood. I was able to slow down and focus on small, incremental changes that set the groundwork for my long and slow process of feeling like myself again. According to Brianna,

> The most common misconception when returning to exercise postpartum is that everybody is ready to return to exercise by their six-week checkup. You may feel like you are "out of the woods" physically, but the reality is your body is still healing. It took your body nine months to adjust to carrying a baby; it may take nine months, if not more, to adjust to your new body. I know no one wants to hear that, but taking into consideration the rapid weight change and shift in center of gravity, how your joints stabilize in space and throughout movement will be affected. Your lumbo-pelvo-hip muscles have also experienced trauma and are in no condition to support high-intensity or long duration exercises. Now, this does not mean you do not exercise. You can begin breath work as early as twenty-four hours after birth. Walking is 100 percent safe and a very good idea. . . . I have had clients "ready" (for the basics) at four weeks; however, every mother, no matter the fitness level, starts with breath and stability work. Regaining the neuromuscular connection to the pelvic floor, core, and glutes is key to setting an optimal foundation for the work ahead.[3]

Exercise may be something that you are dying to get back to, or it may be the last thing on your mind. If you really want to start working out again postpartum, just remember that anything other than light activity such as walks can be detrimental before you are cleared by your provider at six weeks postpartum. I get it—if you are used to working out regularly and it helps you mentally feel good, it can be hard during the stressful postpartum period to do less than you are used to. However, injury may lead to more long-term complications and setbacks.

When returning to exercise, make sure you are doing it in a conscious way. Alignment and technique are very important when working out during the postpartum period. And you will not be where you were prior to giving birth or prior to being pregnant. There are a lot of trainers who specialize in postpartum exercise, but even if you cannot access these resources in person, they often post videos on social media or have websites where you can access basic tips for free. I have included some free vetted resources in the back of this book to get you started. Be wary of those that offer quick results. As Brianna told me, "If someone or a business is promoting fat loss, waist trimming, arm-slimming exercises for the postpartum demographic, you should unfollow. Those movements are likely to spike your cortisol levels and heighten your nervous system, which is not what you need while in recovery or healing. The priority should be intentional connection and support. Can you lift and hold your baby without pain? Not can you do ten burpees in a row."

Both Brianna and Joanie told me that no matter what your exercise regimen prior to delivery, no matter what your level of physical fitness pre-baby, and no matter whether you gave birth vaginally or via cesarean, during the postpartum period, everyone starts with the basics: breathing, learning to connect with your core, and how to brace when picking up the baby. Corrective exercise, which is the study of how your brain connects to your muscles, "is not sexy," Joanie admits. For instance, one of the exercises she gives her clients is getting off the floor. However, mastering basic functional movements prevents pain and injury. Although tedious, they pay off in the long term, as you are able to safely return to the exercises you love. People who have practiced corrective exercise prior to giving birth tend to regain the mind-body connection and pathways much more quickly postpartum, but everyone, no matter their antepartum fitness level, still has to start with the basics.

REHABILITATING YOUR PELVIC FLOOR

Besides finding a trusted perinatal trainer to help guide you in your postpartum recovery, I also highly recommend working with a pelvic floor physical therapist, if possible. Just as with the trainers, working with physical therapists prior to giving birth will help you get back to the basics more quickly. Even if you did not see them pre-baby, when you go to your postpartum visit and are cleared for normal activity, don't forget to ask your provider for a referral to a pelvic floor physical therapist (PT). Perinatal trainers and pelvic floor PTs both agree that the combination of internal and external work really helps in recovery, and these specialists can communicate and better understand what is going on in your body, creating a collaborative plan tailored to you. Pelvic floor physical therapists can assess your pelvic floor internally through vaginal exams, allowing them to directly assess how well you are engaging your pelvic floor muscles and to ascertain any areas of pain, muscle tightness, or muscle relaxation. This can help them provide you feedback, so you know when you are doing the exercises correctly and when you are not. For example, Ronit told me that many people don't have good function and awareness of their pelvic floor muscles and may think that they are contracting them when they are bearing down and vice versa, which can lead to issues like constipation, worsening prolapse, or incontinence. Pelvic floor physical therapists can help you regain your pelvic floor strength and decrease or eliminate incontinence, symptoms from prolapse, or constipation. They can also help with pelvic and perineal pain so that you can be comfortable returning to your usual activities such as exercise and intercourse. Ronit also has worked with clients who thought their chronic pain with penetration was just a normal part of having sex—until she taught them it wasn't and helped them get relief from that pain. We often don't talk about these things freely with our friends and family, so we don't have anything to compare our experience with, making it hard to recognize when something is actually abnormal.

Just as with the experts in perinatal training that I spoke to, she encouraged waiting until being cleared by your provider to resume physical activity, except for basics such as light stretching, walking, and diaphragmatic breathing. She also recommended asking your provider in the hospital to have a physical therapist see you while on postpartum prior to discharge, which is a wonderful pearl of wisdom. Every hospital has physical therapists and occupational therapists who can see patients postoperatively. Although this may not be the case at every birthing facility, your hospital may have someone who can help reinforce the basics, such as how to safely get out of bed and how to go to the bathroom.

WHAT HAPPENED TO MY BELLY?!

I hate to use this term, but as it is the most common part of their post-birth body that new parents ask about and point to in dislike, I feel I need to address the "mom pooch." "Mom pooch" is not fat. It is diastasis recti, the physiologic and aesthetic result of your abdominal muscles stretching, relaxing, and separating in the midline to make space for your growing baby throughout pregnancy. This creates loose skin and muscles in the lower abdomen that is often referred to as a "pooch." Even with a vaginal birth, your rectus muscles separate and stretch due to growing a full human. With a cesarean birth, they must be further separated in the midline during the surgery (except in very rare circumstances, the rectus muscles are not cut) to gain access to the uterus.

You may have stretch marks or you may not, and the linea nigra, or dark line down the middle of your abdomen, won't go away immediately. Stretched skin cannot be "toned." Your skin has only a certain amount of elasticity and may always show signs of the fact that you carried a baby in your belly. The muscle tone improves on its own over time and can improve more rapidly with exercise once you're cleared to work out by your obstetric provider. However, it is important to watch out for diastasis with abdominal or core workouts, as improper technique can put stress on your muscles and lead to further separation.

FOCUS ON HOW YOU FEEL

As you work toward recovering your physical strength and conditioning and getting back to feeling comfortable with your body, it is so important to remember to focus on how you feel more than how you look. Every expert I have spoken to has reiterated this. It is a long journey, typically six months to a year, before their clients are ready to graduate. And they encourage them not to focus on the pounds or the inches, but rather on how their body feels. Success means they are able to do something without pain. They are stronger.

Plan on it being a longer journey, and when you look back after a month or a year, you really will be able to appreciate what you can do that you couldn't do before. It can take much longer than six weeks to even be ready to start working out again. Your body rapidly becomes deconditioned during the time you are inactive or much less active. You also may need to focus on your pain and scarring from birth, as well as other symptoms such as incontinence, before fully focusing on the physical work required to get back in shape. It may be years before you take inventory of yourself and realize that you feel like you again and are able to do the same activities you did before at the same level. This journey is in no way one-size-fits-all. It is not for the faint of heart. It takes time, but with patience, your end goal in mind, and a lot of self-compassion, you will get there.

I really want to reiterate this last point. *You will get there.* According to Joanie, one of the biggest misconceptions her clients have is that "they are going to suffer in some way because of this process. Forever. [They worry] that things are never going to feel normal again. That they are not going to regain full strength. And that's not true. A symptom in your pelvic floor is a symptom that can be addressed. You can love your body again and you can love it even more than you did before."

I could not agree more. My body is not the same body it was before getting pregnant with my first daughter. And it changed again after my second birth. But today, I have much more gratitude and respect for my body, this body that has grown and birthed two human beings and bears signs of those parts of my journey. And now my body is not just feeling love from me. Those two little human beings, which I created with this body, also show it so much love and affection (and yes, occasionally they comment on my soft, stretchy belly, not in criticism but out of appreciation for having a place to rest their little heads when they are tired).

POSTPARTUM NUTRITION

According to Jaz Robbins, psychologist and nutritionist, we must account for a person's baseline health. This is why it is important to work with someone who can do a full assessment and make recommendations based on your individual needs. Just like creating a postpartum exercise plan or infant plan, it is hard to make general recommendations, as everyone's bodies and specific health needs are unique.

That said, her baseline recommendations for postpartum are as follows:

After pregnancy, the focus of nutrition becomes twofold, (1) helping one heal from the strain that the birthing process placed on the body, and (2) helping provide adequate nutrition for those who are nursing their babies. In addition to addressing these concerns, most postnatal vitamin supplements are formulated to also help improve mood and decrease brain fog—more often referred to as "baby brain."

The nutrient that requires the most significant increase from pregnancy to postpartum is vitamin A. For most, their vitamin A requirement shifts from 770 micrograms while pregnant to 1,300 micrograms postpartum. Vitamin A plays a key role in immune function and helps to keep infants healthy as they acclimate to the environment and world around them. Though they will still benefit from a postnatal vitamin, those who are not nursing will not have this increased need for vitamin A.[4]

We know that food deserts are a real issue and not everyone has access to good quality nutrition. That said, Jaz recommends focusing on the small decisions you make when it comes to your diet.

- Make certain to take your prenatal vitamins
- Take advantage of any opportunities to enjoy fresh produce and unprocessed foods
- Hydrate with water and avoid soda and sugary drinks

If you are a family or friend of someone giving birth, instead of buying them cute baby clothes (or in addition to), think about preparing them meals that they can freeze, paying for a month of a meal delivery service (Jaz recommends both MealPro, which has prenatal options, and Kitchen Doula, which offers both pre- and postnatal options), or offering to send them food when you are ordering delivery for yourself.

As ever, show yourself some compassion and remember that your mental health and well-being matters as well. Don't criticize yourself if you eat fast food one day, or if you just can't even think about doing your exercises for the day. Listen to yourself and if you need sleep or a long warm shower more than your Kegels that day, give yourself permission to do what you need without feeling guilty about it.

In the next chapter, we discuss the resumption of other major physical activities after giving birth: sexual intercourse and physical intimacy. This can be a very daunting and complex topic. Just like with exercise and nutrition, your history, birth experience, and personal goals are all very relevant. That said, let's dive into this other topic, which is rarely discussed and prepared for with your healthcare provider or even your partner before or after giving birth. Let's talk about sex!

TWELVE

INTIMACY, SEX, AND FAMILY PLANNING AFTER BABY

When you go to your routine postpartum visit around six weeks after giving birth, your doctor will ask you a few questions about how you and the baby are doing, do a physical exam to make sure you have healed, and clear you to return to normal activities. When I first finished my training as an OB/GYN, the dialogue during these visits tended to focus a lot more on the baby and less on the person who had given birth. Often new parents brought the babies with them to the appointments, so there was an even greater focus on the new little human in the room. After fawning over the baby, I would get to work examining the birth parents and asking about pain, bleeding, bowel and bladder function, mood, and feeding, as well as plans for contraception. I would do a breast and pelvic exam (as well as an abdominal exam if they had a C-section) and then clear them to return to normal activities, including exercise and sex (meaning penetrative intercourse, which, as we all know, does not equate directly to pleasure for both partners—it just means that you can insert a penis or other penetrating object into your vagina). I laugh when I think about this conversation (or really, lack of conversation) now, as sex was the last thing on my mind when I was six weeks postpartum!

When clearing parents to return to normal activities, I give a few important caveats regarding sex:

1. Just because your provider says you can resume having intercourse does not in any way mean that you will want to immediately have sex. There are many reasons, all valid, that a lot of birthing parents are nowhere near ready for sex, especially penetrative sex, only six weeks after birthing a baby.

2. If there was any tearing, there may be scar tissue, which makes it uncomfortable and sometimes painful to resume intercourse initially. Start with perineal massage to get reacquainted with your postpartum body and to soften any tender or tighter areas with scar tissue. With a C-section, there may be internal scar tissue, so deep penetration may be uncomfortable.

3. Besides the physical components, a huge aspect of feeling ready to have sex is mental and emotional. Communicate these needs to your partner and try to get the support you need, whether that is a therapist, a pelvic floor physical therapist, or other resources to help you feel emotionally and mentally ready for intercourse.

4. Intimacy is not just intercourse. There are many ways to be intimate and to show your partner you love them without having sex.

Before going into some of the common reasons you may not feel like having sex, I do want to say that some people cannot wait to start having sex again. Some people really want to reconnect with their partners and their bodies in this way, so they are anxiously waiting to be cleared for sex. If this is you, go for it! The last thing I want to do is alienate people who feel like having sex when they have an infant at home. No matter how you're feeling about sex, there is information in this chapter that will be helpful for you when you do regain that level of intimacy with your partner, so please do not skip this section if you are ready to have sex again!

WHY DON'T I FEEL LIKE HAVING SEX?

Change in Hormones

The drop in estrogen that occurs after giving birth is substantial, and estrogen levels stay low while breastfeeding/chestfeeding. You may have noticed some night sweats and/or hot flashes during the immediate postpartum period, and they may still be occurring even at six weeks. Postpartum estrogen levels are low, just like in menopause. This is because nature does not want you to get pregnant again right away. They will increase again over time, but they do not get back to baseline quickly, especially if you are breastfeeding. Your body is smart—when you are exclusively breast-feeding/chestfeeding, your body knows it's not the best time to get pregnant again. (This does not mean you cannot ovulate while breastfeeding, though, especially as you space the feeds out, so please always use a form of contraception if you do not want to get pregnant again right away!)

Low estrogen also decreases your sex drive and your arousal, which can lead to less lubrication, making penetration uncomfortable or even downright painful. I tell new parents this so that they can be prepared with a good water- or silicone-based lubricant if they do want to resume intercourse. These lubricants also can be used instead of a natural oil for the aforementioned perineal massage. Sometimes the first step to regaining intimacy is having your partner touch and massage you gently so you get a sense for how the vagina and perineum feel after healing. Your partner should understand that lack of lubrication does not equal lack of desire for them or for sex. Part-ners may feel rejected if their partner does not physiologically appear to be "turned on," so they need to respect other verbal and physical cues to know when the birthing person is ready and open and de-siring touch and sex.

Your provider also can prescribe vaginal estrogen for you to help during the postpartum period. This is not only helpful in plumping the tissues and making sex more comfortable, but also in expediting healing if you have any tearing or incontinence after birth. Pelvic floor physical therapists encourage all of their clients working on post-partum recovery to start vaginal estrogen.

Sleep Deprivation

Lack of sleep means sex may be the last thing on your mind. This is very common and it is totally okay to prefer sleep over sex—or literally anything and everything else you can fill your precious time with. When you have a baby, you are in survival mode first, so ba-sics like eating, sleeping, perhaps even taking a shower, will all take priority over sex. Catharine McDonald, an incredible therapist with multiple specialties including sex therapy, recommends that, when you are ready, try to incorporate intimacy earlier in the day before you are completely maxed out and exhausted with the baby.[1] Intimacy does not equate to intercourse, and you can express intimacy in many ways as discussed later.

Feeling "Touched Out"

If you do not feel ready to have intercourse, you can still experience other forms of physical intimacy such as cuddling or massage. However, even this may feel like too much physical contact when you have given birth recently. This is due to all of the physical contact and touch with your baby. You simply may not need or desire the touch of your partner in addition to all of that. You may even recoil from it. The intense bonding and physical contact with your new baby may lead you to feel "touched out." If you have older children as well, they will inevitably want more of your attention and touch to reassure them that they are not forgotten or less important, so you barely may be able to go pee without someone on your lap, let alone get any personal body space during this new baby time.

Breastfeeding or chestfeeding adds another level of touch intensity, as you are not only holding your baby, but they are literally latched onto you throughout the day and night. All of this may lead to a lack of desire for any intimate touch with your partner. You may just fantasize about laying sprawled out in your bed, alone, with no one trying to get a piece of you. As a new mom, I often fantasized about checking into a hotel room by myself far away from the reach of my family. Instead, I used my very brief showers to enjoy a few minutes of peace after my first was born. After the second, even that time was interrupted by a very jealous and insecure four-year-old claiming any of my time that she could when the baby was relegated to a different room. This meant many showers when my little shadow would run in the bathroom, strip off her clothes, and join me.

Infant Bonding and Endorphins

Physical touch from your baby is not all draining, however. It also can be very pleasurable and actually releases a lot of positive endorphins. These endorphins are like a love drug and keep us coming back for more, thus strengthening the bond between parent and infant. As human infants cannot care for themselves like many other animal species, evolution created a system of positive feedback to keep us craving contact and proximity with our babies. This can mean that you don't desire sex or other physical intimacy with your partner because you are fully satiated and filled with the same positive endorphins released from sexual intimacy when you touch your baby's skin, feel their little fingers grasp your own, bend over to inhale their new baby smell, or cover them in kisses. I felt totally fulfilled from a physical intimacy point with both of my babies. Even though at times I wanted to run away by myself for some much-needed personal space, I also really loved the weight of my soft squishy babies against my body and did not desire any other form of physical touch.

Birth Trauma

Birth trauma, whether or not it meets the clinical criteria for post-traumatic stress disorder, is extremely prevalent. Trauma is in the eye of the beholder, so no one else can tell you if your birth experience should or should not have resulted in trauma. Trauma can result from any part of the birth experience in which you did not feel safe or in control of your body. After experiencing a traumatic birth, it can be scary to think about having physical intimacy and sex again. There are so many elements that feed into this. What is triggering and what is necessary to feel safe, trusting, and embodied enough to desire physical intimacy and receive pleasure from it varies greatly depending on your experience and how you perceived and internalized it. For some people, the simple fact that sex led to pregnancy in the first place can make it the last thing you desire. It may also take a while to be ready to start processing your birth experience with a trusted professional.

If your partner is giving you cues that they are ready to be intimate, but you are nowhere near ready for penetrative intercourse, let alone physical touch, how do you let them know without them getting offended? According to psychologist Jaz Robbins,

> [this is an] obstacle that is rooted in the history of your relationship, the trust that has been present in your relationship, and communication (or lack thereof) present in your relationship. It's difficult for anyone to masterfully build a life raft while they're in the process of sinking. It's much more advantageous to build it before you need it. Having this conversation is easiest for couples whose relationships are already resting on a solid foundation of respect, trust, and open communication. Without those elements, birth trauma survivors will find themselves trying to build this foundation during a time when they may feel like they are drowning in the emotional aftermath of their trauma.[2]

Working with a trauma specialist to help process your trauma, as well as a couples therapist to help navigate this time, especially between partners lacking a strong bond of trust, respect, and healthy, honest communication before the birth, can help you both navigate these experiences and even build a stronger bond as a couple. It takes a level of vulnerability between two people to do this work and for most of us that can be really hard, so the more work done before birth, the better dynamic you will have with your partner as you both navigate the aftermath of birth trauma.

And let's not forget partners who were present during the traumatic event and develop secondary trauma from this experience, which they also will need to process. Watching your loved one going through something scary and feeling helpless to do anything for them is extremely hard and may affect their desire to regain physical intimacy as well.

Adjusting to Your Postpartum Body

Besides the changes that occur with perineal tearing or abdominal surgery, the abdominal muscles relax, the breasts change (even if not breastfeeding), and weight changes, none of which resolves right away—or sometimes ever. It is impossible to grow and birth a human, even if you had the easiest delivery and recovery, without having some internal and external physical changes as well as mental and emotional changes.

Coming to a place of comfort and love for your postpartum body is different for everyone. Some people may feel empowered and a new sense of appreciation and love for their body after knowing what it has accomplished. Others, however, may mourn their prepregnancy body and may not feel comfortable being intimate, because they are not comfortable personally with their new physical identity and are not mentally in a space to let someone else see them intimately. Some people return to feeling like they did before and others never do.

Lack of Desire for Your Partner

Let's face it. Having a baby will test your relationship with your partner in ways few other scenarios can. I have heard people say they want to have a baby to save their relationship, but bringing home a baby leads to new stressors, some of which you may have been prepared for, and others that you have never thought of. Add to that sleep deprivation, the 24/7 burden of caring for the baby, and everything else you may be doing to help out around the house, and you may feel more rage than love toward your partner.

Communication also easily breaks down, because when you give birth, your brain literally changes, so you do not think and feel the same way that you did before. My therapist brought this to my attention after the birth of my second child. She said that my partner could not expect me to have the same ability to process things as I had before giving birth. I was recovering from surgery, experiencing massive hormonal shifts, and not sleeping well. I literally wasn't myself, so how we communicated and our expectations around resolving disputes could not remain the same either.

INTIMACY WITHOUT SEX

It is always important to remember that you can still be intimate with your partner without sex. Intimacy involves being vulnerable with someone else, so it can include physical touch that does not lead to sex. When I spoke to Catharine McDonald, she gave this advice:

> If the only time two adults touch each other in ways they don't touch other people is in the moments prior to sex, then I think that the mom's body kind of shuts down and buttons up. It's like, "I know it's coming." Partners need to make sure they're not just touching sensually. Their touch needs to say, "You are my partner, and you are beautiful."

Intimacy also can be purely emotional vulnerability and connection, by being honest and open about how you are feeling, how you are adjusting to parenthood, what you miss about your old life without the baby, what scares you about being a parent. According to Andrew Wheeler, board certified pastoral counselor, and Elizabeth Wheeler, licensed pastoral counselor:

> So much of intimacy actually doesn't have to be sexual at all. Think about other ways that [your] partner sees intimacy, experiences intimacy, or feels a connection of any sort from them aside from sex. If we are able to connect on intimate levels aside from the physical, then it makes the physical side come more natural and feel easier. Being able to normalize any feeling whether you feel ready at the six-week mark or whether you don't even think you can comprehend when you will be ready, those are both normal feelings and experiences postpartum, and every couple is going to be different and every birthing person is going to be different. Being as open with your partner as you possibly can about where you're at, what you're feeling, what you're experiencing, [and] including them in the process can make it easier for the partner to understand and meet you where you're at as well as be patient and understanding.[3]

Getting Professional Support

If your physical recovery has made it difficult for you to think about having and enjoying sex again, then please find a local pelvic floor physical therapist to get evaluated and start the work to improve any residual pain, discomfort, and other physical symptoms such as stress urinary incontinence. You want to feel like yourself again and be in a place where you can enjoy sex. If you have emotional and mental blocks that are holding you back from wanting to have sex, find individual and/or couples therapists that specialize in perinatal support, as well as sex therapists who are competent in this area, to help you with your recovery. If you have trauma to work through that is being triggered by the thought of having intercourse, then a good trauma therapist can help you process it and develop tools to implement when you feel triggered.

Catharine McDonald, whom I mentioned earlier, is a therapist who focuses on the perinatal period and works with a lot of birth people and their partners during pregnancy and after birth. She reminds her pregnant and postpartum clients that "setting expectations with partners will result in really amazing sex when you are ready. Returning to intimacy takes time, and there's going to be an uphill climb. Giving birth, no matter which way a baby comes out, changes how things feel. You have to figure out what feels good, and then you've got to communicate that to your partner."

So how do you start to refamiliarize yourself with your postpartum body, learn what feels good and what doesn't now, and feel comfortable with allowing your partner to explore your body again? Catharine recommends self-exploration: "Touch your body while you're cleaning yourself in the shower or bath. Use a gentle soap or coconut oil to reduce friction. You're not being watched; no one's waiting to see if it leads to more. Real-time feedback in the safety of a private space helps avoid the painful experience."

Sex in general is something that we often feel pressured to engage in, and sometimes people end up having sex before they feel ready because their partner is pressuring them or they feel the societal pressure that they "should" want to have sex, otherwise there is something wrong with them or their relationship with their partner. As Catharine muses, "how the partner responds [to the conversation around resuming intercourse] is really predictive of how well it will go for the next year and beyond. If a partner is nurturing and patient, checking in with the birth parent, and truly partnering, that can be incredibly beautiful"—and can lead to even better sex down the road.

Desire for sex and physical intimacy looks different for every person, even prior to giving birth. Postpartum, I encourage you to listen to yourself and your body and not try to push yourself into a situation that makes you feel uncomfortable or in which you don't feel good. Communicate with your partner about how you are feeling so they understand this is not a personal rejection. Despite all of the reasons you may not currently feel like having sex, for most people who desired physical intimacy prior to having a baby, time eventually resolves these blocks and you will desire sex and other acts of physical intimacy again. Please make sure you keep reading so you are ready when that time comes!

OVULATION AND FERTILITY POSTPARTUM

This section is specifically relevant to those who are having heterosexual intercourse and who have the physiologic possibility of conceiving with intercourse (for example, your partner does not have azoospermia, or your fallopian tubes have not been removed). Ovulation will happen before you have your first period, so if you don't want to get pregnant again right away, use a reliable method of birth control. Even if you are exclusively breastfeeding/chestfeeding, you may start to ovulate again without realizing it as the feeds space out.

Even with a history of infertility of unknown cause or related to hormonal imbalances, such as polycystic ovarian syndrome, don't assume that you cannot get pregnant after giving birth. Unless your fertility specialist has told you that you physically cannot conceive without assisted reproductive technology, do not assume that you cannot get pregnant. I have had many patients who experienced years of infertility prior to having their baby and then return, dumbfounded, when they get pregnant again when the baby is only a few months old. Their body reset and their fertility improved. Or maybe it was just the lack of stress and pressure from trying to get pregnant and now that they've had a baby, that stress is gone. Needless to say, don't assume you aren't fertile unless there is a known, definitive reason that you or your partner cannot get pregnant without assisted reproductive technology.

CONTRACEPTION

Some new moms are eager to have an IUD placed, have their tubes tied, or get their partner to the urologist for a vasectomy. Other new moms have had side effects with birth control and are avidly opposed or just have never used birth control and prefer to stay off of it. For those of you interested in all of your family planning options, this section covers the basics of different options so that you feel confident having this discussion with your provider. Even if you feel rushed at your postpartum visit, you can be prepared with an answer to the question, "Are you interested in starting birth control?" after reading this section. I want you to feel empowered to make an educated, person-centered decision based on your family planning goals and your body. One of my favorite sites for information about all of your contraception options is Bedsider (https://www.bedsider.org). It includes not only easy-to-read information on all methods, including the most recent data and statistics, but it also offers patient testimonials and many other educational posts related to all things family planning. I recommend referring to this site after reading the rest of this chapter to get more information on each specific method, as a comprehensive discussion of contraception is beyond the scope of this book. The following is a brief overview of how I talk to my patients about contraception methods.

Temporary Contraception Methods

Temporary methods can be divided into categories a few different ways. The most common ways I look at them and review them with my patients are hormonal versus nonhormonal and short acting versus long acting.

If you are breastfeeding, a nonhormonal or progesterone-only method is usually recommended, because combined hormonal methods with estrogen may decrease your milk supply. Hormonal methods also can cause other side effects such as mood changes, bloating, headaches, skin changes, and, with estrogen, the rare but serious side effect of blood clots if you are at higher risk of blood clots in your legs or lungs. Whether the method has only progesterone or progesterone and estrogen, the type of progesterone, the amount of hormones, as well as whether the method is locally acting or systemic (released locally from inside the vagina or uterus versus being absorbed in the bloodstream by oral ingestion or through the skin/subdermal) also affects how your body will metabolize it.

Single-use methods must be used every time you have intercourse. Condoms, spermicide, and Phexxi are examples. Short-acting methods are single use or ones that you must use regularly on a daily or weekly basis to be effective. The pill, the patch, and the vaginal ring are part of this category. Medroxyprogesterone, the intramuscular injection, lasts for around three months. Long-acting reversible contraceptives are devices inside the uterus or under the skin that last for anywhere from three to ten years. All intrauterine devices and the subdermal implant Nexplanon are part of this category.

Single-use and short-term methods require you to remember to take them or use them, so their efficacy, or proper use, tends to be lower, meaning that unintended pregnancy rates will be higher. Long-term methods are inserted and removed by a provider; however, their efficacy is much higher (put in and forget it), since you don't have to remember to do anything for them to stay effective (except remove them when they expire). Medroxyprogesterone is also considered very efficacious since it is a one-time injection every three months and there is less chance for user error. Long-acting reversible methods (meaning not permanent) are considered to be cost effective

---

NONHORMONAL VERSUS HORMONAL CONTRACEPTIVES

Nonhormonal: condoms, Phexxi, copper intrauterine device (IUD)
Hormonal:
- progesterone only: mini pill (norethindrone), subdermal implant (Nexplanon), medroxyprogesterone, and progesterone IUDs
- estrogen and progesterone: combined oral contraceptive pills, vaginal ring, birth control patch

if you plan to use them for at least a year. If you plan on trying to get pregnant again rather quickly or really don't think you want to be on birth control for at least a year, then a short-term method may be better for you.

Permanent Contraception Methods

There are two permanent methods for avoiding pregnancy: sterilization via bilateral tubal ligation or bilateral salpingectomy and vasectomy.

These methods are meant to be nonreversible. If you are interested in a tubal ligation (now more commonly a bilateral salpingectomy is performed, which is the complete removal of the fallopian tubes), make sure you know the rules in your state. Consent forms often have to be signed in advance of the procedure (in New York, thirty days prior to delivery if delivering full term or seventy-two hours prior to preterm delivery). This is meant to prevent coercion at the time of the birth. Even if you don't anticipate having a C-section, it is always good to have this paperwork on file in advance so if you end up needing a C-section, the tubal ligation can be performed at the same time. It adds minimal time and risk to the procedure and is much easier than going back for another surgery under general anesthesia at a later date.

Some hospitals and physicians also offer immediate postpartum bilateral tubal ligation prior to hospital discharge for those who have had a vaginal birth. However, this is not universal practice due to availability of operating rooms and physicians, so it's always good to think about whether you may be interested in this. Otherwise, tubal ligation can be done as soon as six weeks postpartum via laparoscopic surgery once the uterus has involuted (returned to its normal size).

A vasectomy for your partner can be done at any point as an outpatient procedure under local anesthesia. For anyone who desires permanent sterilization and is in a long-term, stable relationship with a male partner, the option for male sterilization is always great to discuss, as it entails less risk than surgery under general or regional anesthesia.

So that's it. We made it through some of the most uncomfortable and yet important topics in this chapter. In the coming chapters, we explore some of the less visible aspects of becoming a new parent: your changing self-identity and how you can get the support and time you need to thrive during this crazy period of your life. No matter how "easy" your baby is, having a new baby is hard. While you figure out the role of parent and who you are now, you deserve the help and support needed to make it through without being completely depleted. The sooner you start to think about that and practice the skills necessary to get what you need, the better you will get at it—so let's get started!

PART III

Matrescence

THIRTEEN

THE MYTHS OF MOTHERHOOD

When I became a mom, I spent the first year working overtime to do everything I thought I had to—I went back to work as soon as I could, I spent long nights with the baby, I worked hard to make sure my house was as tidy as possible. I bent over backward to try to fit the image in my mind of the "ideal mother."

We all have an image such as this in our minds. Yours may not look like mine; you might envision that the ideal mother stays home and homeschools her kids or serves her community continually. All of these images have been acquired from the different cultures, societies, movies, and media surrounding us. In fact, there are four primary images of motherhood specific to the culture that I—and most of us in the United States—have been exposed to throughout our lives: the martyr, the goddess, the superwoman, and the homemaker.

In this chapter, I break down each of these faux ideals, explaining why they're actually impossible standards to meet. These unattainable archetypes leave new moms striving for an ideal standard that just doesn't exist, often losing themselves and what really makes them happy in the process. Once I gave myself permission to stop trying to live up to these myths and worrying about the judgment of others, I became the best type of mom I could be. I learned to love myself as much as I loved my baby and could focus on being present with her and enjoying our time together. Here's what I want you to know—the simple yet very important lesson I had to learn in those early years: you're already a great mom, regardless of what society and media depict.

Before getting into the myths of motherhood, I think it is very important to recognize that not everyone who gives birth identifies as a mother. And not every partner of the birthing person identifies as a father. This, once again, is another instance for which we lack adequate language. Many members of the LGBTQ+ community are creating new terms and finding ways to relate to parenthood that do not involve the traditional terms and the myths that go along with them. However, this, in itself, also can be alienating and feel very isolating. Although more and more people who do not identify as female are giving birth or becoming parents through other means, and more trans men are carrying pregnancies and giving birth, this is still a marginalized community, so I always encourage my patients and friends who identify in nontraditional ways or are in nontraditional partnerships to join support groups specifically for LGBTQ+ parents and also to consider individual and/or couples therapists as they go through pregnancy and transition to parenthood.

For this chapter, I use the terms "mom" and "motherhood" because the myths we're discussing revolve around traditional gender norms and the stereotypes and cultural ideals we place around those who fulfill these roles. If you do not identify as female or as a mother, please take this for what it is and help us destroy these myths in your own way. I hope that during the rest of my years of doing this work, we are able to continue dismantling more of the boxes we try to shove people into along their reproductive and parenthood journeys.

THE MYTHS OF MOTHERHOOD

Society and cultures have created many myths surrounding motherhood, all of which place women into differentiated boxes and teach them that if they do not live up to these standards, they are not a good enough mother. Shari Thurer recognizes this dilemma and writes in her book *The Myths of Motherhood: How Culture Reinvents the Good Mother*:

> The current ideology of good mothering is not only spurious, it is oblivious of a mother's desires, limitations, and context, and when things go wrong, she tends to get blamed. This has resulted in a level of confusion and self-consciousness among mothers that their predecessors never

knew. There is a glaring need to restore to mother her own presence, to understand that she is a person, not merely an object for her child, to recognize her subjectivity.[1]

Some of the most common myths I have encountered follow. They are reinforced by the parts of ourselves that we often project on social media. There is even a whole generation of mommy influencers now who give us more standards to live up to.

The Selfless Martyr Myth

Many moms and moms-to-be unwittingly fall for the image of mom as martyr: the idea that the minute you decide you want to get pregnant, you must become selfless. *Everything* in your life now comes second to the needs, desires, schedules, and stuff of your children. In many cultures this is even applauded and expected of women. I have met countless moms who seem to erase their own individual identities as they slowly give up things they had loved in their lives and replace it all with being moms. Every conversation revolves around their children, and they begin to even forget what they were passionate about before kids.

Of course, we all make some compromises as we weigh what is most important to us and determine how children fit into our lives without completely consuming them. Rather than losing ourselves, let's become self-fulfilled, for only when we have filled ourselves will we have enough energy and capacity to physically, mentally, emotionally, and spiritually care for a baby. No one is meant to lose themselves completely when they become a mother.

Being a mom is a role we play at a certain time in our lives. When you give yourself completely to this role and dedicate yourself entirely to the tasks of raising children, you not only miss out on a lot of the joy that comes from being your own complete person and teaching your children how to follow their own dreams, love themselves, and take care of themselves, but you also open yourself up to the suffering that can occur once your children are grown and leave the home. If your life revolves completely around serving them, who are you once they no longer require your full devotion and energy? Who are you as a person, a partner, and a friend? You will have lost your identity and your life force in the temporary role you fulfilled.

This does not mean that I think parents should not be stay-at-home parents or sacrifice for their children in other ways—this is the hardest job in the world. Raising good human beings and doing it in a conscious way is a task that requires much dedication and hard work. But it should not require full and complete self-sacrifice. No matter what imagery you see from cultural and religious stereotypes, parents are people, too, and just as you want your children to find their own course and pursue their own passions, they want to see you setting that example by living fully as well.

The Goddess Myth

These are the moms we see on social media, posing in their pregnancy and newborn photos with flowy dresses, long wavy hair, and smiles on their faces as they look down serenely and lovingly at their baby bumps or infants. They seem to emanate the idea that they were made for the role of motherhood and are transitioning into parenthood effortlessly and looking amazing while doing so. Some women are naturally physically beautiful by societal standards, effervescent, and literally glow when pregnant and after having a baby. But most women do not look or feel like a goddess when pregnant or after having a baby. Some of us still try to create that picture-perfect image for our pregnancy and infant photo shoots and make sure that every post on social media reinforces this image. We try to convey that we are always happy and blissful, enjoying every stage of the pregnancy, from birth, postpartum recovery, through infancy.

For those of you who do not feel or look this way, please know that most women do not feel amazing during pregnancy. They may be filled with joy or they may not be. But most still have one or more of the following symptoms during pregnancy: vomiting, reflux, constipation, bloating, back pain, pelvic pain, rib pain, swelling, and leg cramps. They feel fat. They are exhausted. Although some women have glowing skin, many develop acne or other skin conditions such as eczema, melasma, and stretch marks. They are sleep deprived (yes, even during the pregnancy) and they are irritable. Some women really just do not like how they look and feel while being pregnant. They miss their old bodies and may even become resentful of their partners for not having to undergo the physical and biochemical changes that are associated with growing a baby. This, of course, may then lead to guilt, especially if this was a highly desired pregnancy, as the mom judges herself poorly for feeling this way. Society tells her that she should not feel bad or upset or annoyed; she should feel blissful and share her natural radiance and glow with everyone around her. The truth is that you don't have to be happy all of the time during pregnancy. This does not make you a bad mom. It is 100 percent okay if you don't feel amazing during your pregnancy.

During postpartum recovery, a whole other set of physical, mental, and emotional changes set in. Needless to say, when your vagina and labia are swollen and painful or your abdomen was just cut open, and you're experiencing things like incontinence, lack of regular showers, painful cracked nipples, and engorgement if you are breastfeeding, it is normal not to feel like a goddess. Some women are very good at embracing all of this messiness and accepting that this is the reality of postpartum life for the majority of us. Some of us feel really bad about ourselves if we cannot live up to the goddess myth. Some, like me, feel disconnected from their new bodies altogether. I would stare at myself in the mirror and not recognize the person in the reflection at all. For both of my postpartum experiences, I did not feel fully like myself again until around the one-year postpartum mark.

I scheduled newborn photos a week after my first daughter was born, and I was mentally miserable and physically still in a lot of pain from my C-section. I had to stop crying and make sure my eyes were not puffy and red when the photographer arrived. But I kept the photography appointment as scheduled, and in the photos, it looked like everything was going beautifully. I still have some of the photos, but I display only the ones of my babies that I know reflect the reality rather than the false images of me that were created that day. I feel sad when I look at that seemingly happy version of myself and think about how hard I struggled before getting the support that I needed.

No matter where you fall on the spectrum during pregnancy and postpartum, you are right where you should be. Just as at any other time, please try to remember that how someone looks in pictures or when you see them out in public is just a snapshot in time. Try not to compare yourself to other moms and just be you.

The Superwoman Myth

Every parent is already superhuman. But no one can live up to the standards of the superwoman who can do it all and do it all perfectly. Especially for those of us who are used to being type A perfectionists, you may have envisioned a life where you seamlessly returned to your job, even a mere six to twelve weeks postpartum, and were able to work with the same energy and priorities as before, then transition to home life, where you cook, clean, and take care of your children, while ensuring that all of their activities are organized and without missing a single milestone. You would then change into your sexy lingerie after the baby was asleep and play your third role—that of the sexy lover—when your partner came home. Oh, and let's not forget the girl's weekends, brunches with friends, nights out, and mom play-dates, all of which you would be able to incorporate flawlessly into your schedule. I am exhausted just typing all of this.

My goal post-child has become figuring out the best work-life balance for me and my family so I still feel like myself and am able to pursue my passions, but also able to be a good mom (not the "best") and not feel guilty when I go to work out or meet a friend for dinner. This balance continually evolves, but I have learned to live by my values and not for the validation of others, so saying "no" without feeling bad about myself has become an important skill I have developed.

The Perfect Homemaker

This myth tells us that the ideal mom cooks and bakes everything from scratch without ever staining her clothes. She has a spotless home, which is tastefully decorated; she creates beautiful arts and crafts projects and throws the best birthday parties. She also hosts playdates, heads the PTA, and navigates the calendar of events for all of her children seamlessly. She is like the perfect 1950s housewife—except she does not smoke or walk around with a martini every evening (okay, maybe the occasional glass of wine). She may or may not work, but her career is always secondary to her amazing mom and wife skills.

I used to strive to have my house in order every time I had guests over. I never claimed to be a cook, but I prepared hors d'oeuvres and offered sparkling water and cocktails. But now I know that the people who love me will not love me less if the house is not perfect. My kids have turned portions of our apartment into unorganized play zones, and the mess regularly extends throughout the rest of our home on days when they play inside. I have learned that keeping up appearances in my home does not necessarily make me more fulfilled; it just makes me feel that others will judge me more favorably as a "good mom." And because the judgment of others is something I now no longer worry about, I have freed up some time to do things I really want to spend my time doing, like writing this book.

If you get joy from these things, please do them. But really assess the underlying reasons: Are you fulfilling an archetype? Are you making up for where your own mother may have been lacking or trying to live up to the ideal that she set for you? Will you or your kids lead a life that is lacking if you spend some of the energy you use on being the perfect mom, wife, and hostess to do something else that you enjoy even more, like your own hobby, meeting a friend, reading a good book, or just soaking in the tub?

THE BEST MOM IS A REAL MOM

There is no "perfect" pregnancy, "perfect" mom, or "perfect" baby. There is life. Life is dynamic, random, unpredictable, and often messy, scary, and tragic. It is also beautiful, awe-inspiring, and miraculous. Creating new life forces us to confront our complete and utter inability to predict or control the outcomes of our journey. We learn about fragility, vulnerability, and bravery in a whole new way. We all do it differently, and when we see other moms, whether those intimately known to us, strangers on the street, or celebrities on social media, remember that they also have their own journeys. We should support and not judge them, but also not compare ourselves to the version of their life that they chose to share with us. We should not aim to be the martyr, the goddess, the superwoman, or the perfect homemaker. We are not archetypes or stereotypes. We are all unique human individuals with values, goals, and desires. None of us is perfect. Some of us will love being a mom more than others. Some of us will want to stay at home full time with our babies, and some of us will feel the desire to return to work full time or need to do so for economic reasons. We all have different styles of parenting and coping with stress and struggles. We all have different relationships with other members of our family, community, and other support systems.

There are more voices than ever before sharing and embracing aspects of their journey that do not align with societal norms and standards. I applaud everyone who has had the courage to share and become vulnerable. I encourage everyone looking to social media and their community to determine what a "good" conception, pregnancy, birth, postpartum period, and motherhood experience should look like to remember that just like in other areas, many people share only the beautiful, happy, ideal version of themselves when in public and on social media to gain approval, fit in, and feel validated. When things are not going so well or the reality does not meet with your set expectations, realize that many of our expectations around the transition to motherhood are unrealistic because we do not have control over the outcomes.

This is why it's crucial to take care of ourselves. No matter what this journey brings and what you encounter, at the end of the day if you know who you are and what you value most, then you will be able to rise to the challenges of parenthood. In the next chapter, I focus on prioritizing yourself. It may sound impossible during this time, but taking care of yourself is so important not just for you to thrive, but for your baby as well.

FOURTEEN

PRIORITIZING YOURSELF

I see the same story play out over and over when meeting newly postpartum patients for an initial mental health consult. They are white-knuckling it, doing their best to hold it together in front of everyone else, when in reality they are so sleep deprived it's amazing they can form a sentence. They are forcing themselves to breastfeed and pump every few hours around the clock because they feel they "should" do it, but they are miserable. They are not getting any joy from their experience as new parents. Instead of taking care of their own needs, they spend their free moments doing tasks around the home to keep it running while getting frustrated that their partners don't understand how to be helpful or won't do household tasks to their standards. The resentment builds, and they take on more and more. They relentlessly push forward, trying to appear like everything is okay while becoming so exhausted from the effort of maintaining their placid exterior. They are mentally falling apart, physically more drained and depleted than they ever knew possible.

Why do we keep doing this to ourselves? Why don't we focus on self-care and our own health and wellness? And what does that even mean or look like during the postpartum period?

Oxford English Dictionary defines self-care as "the practice of taking action to preserve or improve one's own health," as well as "the practice of taking an active role in protecting one's own well-being and happiness, in particular during periods of stress." As you can see, self-care is any intentional action you take to care for your personal health *and* your well-being. This is a vital skill for birth parents and their partners, and in this chapter, I want to help you learn the skills you need to truly care for yourselves.

REAL WELLNESS AND SELF-CARE

Your wellness is not just physical. In 2006, Margaret Swarbrick published a new approach to mental wellness for mental health providers, which includes eight defined aspects of wellness: physical, emotional, spiritual, social, intellectual, environmental, financial, and occupational. According to Swarbrick, "Wellness is a conscious, deliberate process that requires a person to become aware of and make choices for a more satisfying lifestyle. Wellness is not something that can be commoditized. It is a very individual practice, taking into account your goals, preferences, interests, and strengths."[1]

It can be helpful to define what this means to you prior to giving birth so you can start to create the structure and support system needed to achieve these goals. It can be very easy to lose yourself and feel unable to advocate for your needs when you are caring for your new baby, so try to write down your goals and priorities and keep them close at hand so you can remind yourself of them when you are in the weeds. Communicate these to your partner. Make a plan with your support system so that you will feel empowered to stick to it when you become overwhelmed. This will help to anchor you and remind you to take care of yourself and achieve a better state of personal wellness once the baby comes.

I know this is not easy, and I want to acknowledge that many birthing people can't even fathom thinking about their own needs when they are struggling to maintain adequate housing, financial stability, food, and other basic human necessities for survival. We need social structures in place so that all families can bring home their new babies into a safe and healthy environment. We know this is the bare minimum for the birth parent and the infant to thrive and create a secure bond without the stress and worry of surviving daily life. I applaud the many organizations and activists who work tirelessly within their communities to provide these basic necessities to individuals and who lobby their officials to make these necessities a basic human right. As those of us who work in the mental health space know all too well, our patients cannot even begin to focus on their own mental health and emotional well-being until they feel safe and secure in having the daily basic needs of life met.

Even for those of us lucky enough to have our basic needs met, many people laugh at the idea of self-care during the postpartum period, as they cannot fathom taking any time or energy to focus on their personal health and well-being. However, self-care is not just pampering yourself with grandiose, time-consuming gestures. According to Pooja Lakshmin, MD, reproductive psychiatrist and author of *Real Self-Care (Crystals, Cleanses, and Bubble Baths Not Included)*, real self-care is "an ongoing internal process that guides us toward profound emotional wellness and reimagines how we interact with others. It requires self-knowledge, self-compassion, and ultimately, the willingness to make difficult decisions."[2]

Dr. Lakshmin defines the four key aspects of real self-care as:

1. Setting boundaries and moving past guilt
2. Treating yourself with compassion
3. Becoming closer to your authentic self
4. Asserting your power

Self-care requires you to be "selfish" (a word that we need to reclaim as something good and healthy). It means doing what aligns with your values, needs, and wants, even if that means disappointing or upsetting others. You are just as deserving of your own time and energy as your baby, your partner, your family, your friends, and your colleagues. And only when you embody this philosophy, making yourself a priority in your own life, can you truly show up for everyone else in your life as well.

HOW TO PRIORITIZE YOURSELF

In theory it may sound great, but how can this possibly happen during the postpartum period? Often after having a baby, it seems impossible to do anything for oneself. Even taking a shower, preparing a meal, or getting more than a few hours of sleep becomes nearly impossible. Early parenthood puts us into survival mode. However, it is important not to put your own needs last, as the list of things you need to do or "should" do always grows. You will never be able to check everything off the list. Healthy, thriving birth parents mean healthy, thriving babies, families, and communities, so anything you can do to uplift and care for yourself has benefits that reach much further than doing the dishes.

In many cultures around the world, birth parents are cared for by their mothers, mothers-in-law, or close members of their community. There is a designated period of time, often forty days (approximately equal to the first six weeks postpartum), when they are fed nourishing foods and special drinks to help with healing and lactation. Their hair and body are massaged with oils. They are expected not to leave the house and to focus on themselves and getting to know their new baby. They are expected to replenish themselves, recover from birth, and bond with their baby, relinquishing all other responsibilities not directly related to these goals. Self-care is expected and encouraged.

Here are a few things I tell my patients and friends when discussing the importance of prioritizing themselves during the postpartum period:

1. Know that good enough *is* good enough and that some things on your to-do list can be delegated or deprioritized to make time for you.
2. Be flexible with your prebirth plans for postpartum. If something is not working for you and/or your baby, it is always okay to modify your plan (or completely throw it away and create a new plan that better serves your family).
3. Taking care of yourself and filling your cup is something that you are doing not only for yourself, but also for your baby and your whole family. You are the center of your baby's universe, and their well-being is intrinsically tied to your own. They thrive when you thrive.

During the postpartum period, sleep, nourishment, hydration, and allowing yourself to heal from birth are all nonnegotiables in taking care of yourself. As I have discussed before, sleep is a necessity, and without it you will not be able to function physically, mentally, or emotionally. Whatever else you do or do not do during the day, prioritizing sleep is crucial to survival in the early stages of parenthood. It may seem impossible to eat throughout the day, or even to stop to drink a glass of water. I recommend new parents keep a "survival pack" wherever they tend to feed the baby. Granola bars and other easy-to-grab snacks with protein and calories can be left there along with a big water bottle. Whether breastfeeding or bottle feeding, you will get the hang of supporting the baby with one hand so that you can multitask and use your free hand to feed yourself.

Whether you had a vaginal birth or a cesarean birth, your body needs to heal. Trying to do too much too soon can interfere with healing and even cause damage to your body. I have seen many birth parents squat to pick up a toddler and have their sutures suddenly pop out. Trust me, you do not want to feel the pain of a reopened perineal wound. Remind yourself, and everyone else around you, that you need to spend a lot of time resting in bed or in a comfortable seat without doing anything overly strenuous, especially in the early days and weeks. Other things can be tasked out to those around you or just left undone for a while. Remember: good enough is good enough.

ASKING FOR HELP

If you are like me, you were taught that asking for help is a sign of weakness. Doing it all on my own meant that I was winning at life. After nearly losing my sanity from trying to do it all, I had to retrain my mind to understand that asking for help is a sign of a very insightful person who cares about their own well-being as much as they care about the well-being of everyone around them.

Once I started asking for help, I learned how much my support system wanted to help. They wanted to be useful. Often they just didn't know what needed to be done or couldn't anticipate my needs. And once I started asking for help and delegating tasks, the easier it became. I am now a master delegator and enlist as many people as I can to help make sure I can function as a full human being without drowning in the to-do list of parenthood.

As a new parent, it is so important to learn to ask for help and let others know your boundaries. I hear from new moms who are exhausted and frustrated from doing everything themselves. They expect their support system to instinctively know what needs to be done when often tasks need to be delegated.

I give actionable advice for loved ones so they can step up and be of better service to the birth parent (physically and mentally) during this time; however, of equal importance, I teach birth parents how to ask for help. I help my patients create lists of tasks that can be taken off their plate, learn to share nighttime duties, and also tell their loved ones what is *not* helpful. Additionally, some people in your circle, whether family, friends, or colleagues, may impose upon you and invite themselves over. New birth parents sometimes feel so guilty telling their in-laws or close friends that they cannot come over or setting limits on visiting hours and touching or holding the baby. Guilt should not dictate your boundaries during the postpartum period. This is the time to empower yourself to say what *you* need. Stressing yourself out so that others get what they want from you and your baby is not okay.

SETTING BOUNDARIES

The next most important thing I learned how to do was to say no to requests when it was not something that I wanted or needed to do. I set boundaries. I protected my time. I previously had been a people pleaser and often said yes without thinking, wanting to make everyone else happy and getting a lot of validation about being the person who colleagues and friends turned to. This involved everything from getting dinner with friends to joining a committee at work. And just like asking for help, I learned that the more I said no, the more boundaries I set, the easier it became. I did not become worthless in my professional life or lose friends in my personal life by saying no. I actually became better at everything I did because I wasn't extended beyond my bandwidth and annoyed that I was doing something I really didn't want to do. It's true—you may disappoint people at times—but it is also important that you don't disappoint yourself.

Take inventory of what really matters to you, what you really want to do, and when you feel tempted to do something because you "should." If guilt or shame creep in when you want to find a way to avoid saying yes, then pause to see where those feelings are coming from. Often you will find it is fear of rejection or of feeling less valuable to others. However, our value is not tied to how much we overextend ourselves to please others.

ENLISTING YOUR PARTNER

Prior to delivery, it can be very helpful to discuss who will be among your immediate support system and who will be delegated which tasks primarily. The birth parent will need to focus on recovery, bonding with the baby, and feeding the baby. We've already discussed all of the intense changes that will be going on in the birth parent's body and mind. Imagine how difficult it is to form a complete thought, let alone communicate effectively, when overwhelmed and sleep deprived. Conversations you have about who will be responsible for what and any task lists that you can make in advance will be very helpful.

When I spoke to couples therapist Tracy Torelli, a therapist, educator, and women's mental health specialist, she said this about task delegation in families:

> Couples want to have kids together and want it to be equal, but they don't realize that when they add that kid, they're probably going to more mimic what you grew up in, especially if they feel like they had good parents. So I'll ask a lot of questions like, "In the house you grew up in, if a baby's diaper is dirty and your mom and dad are both in the room, what happens next?" Or if a baby cries in the middle of the night, what happens next? So just trying to get them to recognize that when there are unfamiliar circumstances, they're going to probably do more mimicry than reinvention of the wheel.[3]

In Eve Rodsky's book *Fair Play: A Game-Changing Solution for When You Have Too Much to Do (and More Life to Live)*, the author describes the concept of mental load, which is involved with every task on our to-do list. The mental load is all of the thinking, worrying, and planning that goes into completing each task. When you ask your partner to take over a task, they must take over all aspects of the task, not just the final step of carrying it out. For instance, preparing dinner does not mean just cooking the dinner. It means picking out the menu, seeing what items you need from the grocery store, shopping for those items, and making time in your schedule to actually cook the meal. In heterosexual couples, the majority of the mental load falls on the female partner in the relationship. In same-sex couples, it often falls on the partner who financially contributes less. The companion card deck to *Fair Play* provides an easy way to start a conversation with your partner about who will be responsible for each task and the mental load associated with it.

Just in case I haven't made it clear enough yet, your brain will be different during the postpartum period. Decreasing your mental load and minimizing your to-do list after giving birth is extremely important to maintaining your sanity and to avoid becoming a shell of a human being. Delegation is also very important, as resentment and anger toward your partner can quickly build in the postpartum period. I have heard from countless postpartum birthing parents who are filled with indignation and resentment that their partners are not doing their fair share of the work. They lament that their partners don't know what needs to be done, and when they do take over a task, they don't do it as efficiently or as well as birthing parents themselves would do it. Learning to let someone else do the task even if it isn't done the way you would do it or as quickly as you would be able to do it is so important. Repeat the mantra "good enough is good enough" to yourself when struggling with handing over tasks to your partner and support system.

Communication and understanding between partners can become strained during the postpartum period. Understand that besides the added stressors a new baby brings to your relationship and your daily life, your changing hormones after giving birth also can make it more difficult to communicate as you typically would with your partner. As couples therapists (and a married couple and parents themselves) Beth and Andrew Wheeler told me:

Understanding the hormonal changes that are still going on within [the birth parent] and that will continue to be going on for longer than they may realize can be incredibly helpful. Helping both partners to be mindful and aware of the emotions and the interactions that may feel heightened or may feel out of the ordinary for what they're used to in their dynamic or in their relationship. Remember that it is temporary and that it will level out in time, but in the meantime to continue to communicate every day on what each other is experiencing and how they can best be supporting each other through those experiences.[4]

Postpartum rage can even develop, which is a very common symptom of postpartum depression. Sleep deprivation and burnout can lead to irritability, anger, and rage. The associated emotional outbursts are often directed at the partner. This then leads to feelings of guilt and shame, as the birth parent often does not understand why they have these feelings. When you think about all of the physical and emotional changes you are undergoing, please be gentle with yourself and help your partner understand what you are feeling and what is going on internally to lead to these intense reactions.

MANAGING VISITORS

Visitors should also be given things they can help with, whether bringing meals that can be stored in the freezer, cleaning and doing laundry, and watching the baby so parents can nap, get coffee, shower, or do anything else that makes them feel more like a human with their own needs and desires.

Remember, though: you should never feel like you have to agree to have someone come over to meet the baby or to see you if you do not feel ready, if you are too overwhelmed, or if the visitor will add more stress or bring other negative energy into your environment. I have had patients who were extremely anxious or depressed because a family member came for an extended stay, sometimes imposing themselves directly on the new family or sometimes because their partner did not have the heart to tell their mother that she could not stay with them. The birth parent is the most important person in the home and they must feel comfortable and respected. It is the job of their partner to speak up for them if they can't do it themselves and to help them set boundaries and say no to visitors who cause more stress than they alleviate. This is your home and your baby and no one has jurisdiction over either of you, not even your own mother who gave birth to you once upon a time. She had her time, and as wonderful as being a grandparent may be, it is now her turn to be empathetic and patiently await the right time to get to know her new grandchild.

Knowing when to surround yourselves with your community is just as important as knowing when you need time without visitors, and in the next chapter, we discuss the power and importance of community—the right community—during your postpartum period. Human connection is vital, and we discuss how to engage in your community in ways that are beneficial to your well-being, as well as how to create new communities with other parents.

FIFTEEN

BUILDING YOUR COMMUNITY

Living and practicing in New York, I have cared for and met people from all over the world. Many of them are shocked by the lack of support for new parents in such a developed country. Because there is no real infrastructure in place to support new parents, they often feel isolated and alone, stressed about returning to work a mere two to six weeks after their baby is born and lacking affordable childcare for when they do return to work. They also often comment on the striking difference between the community support they witness in their home cultures versus in the United States.

In the United States, it is common for new parents to return home without nearby family or friends on whom they can rely to help out or simply to commiserate with when they're struggling. This disparity grew even worse during the COVID-19 pandemic. Americans often pride themselves on their independence and autonomy, but during the postpartum period, having a support network is critical.

In the prior chapter, we discussed how to ask for help from those in your trusted support network to help you navigate postpartum life without depleting yourself by doing everything on your own. However, emotional support is also so important in the early days of parenthood. It is important to have your community of those you can talk to without filters in place. People you can truly connect with and talk about those aspects of your experience that do not align with the picture-perfect image projected in society. We need a village that validates our experiences and feelings as new parents. This chapter discusses how to engage those already among your trusted network as well as how to put yourself out there to meet new friends who have kids—especially if you're one of the first in your circle to have a baby.

IT TAKES A VILLAGE

Most of you have heard the phrase, "It takes a village." As an American who has always been very independent and self-sufficient, I never appreciated this phrase until I had my first baby. Having supportive family, friends, and colleagues can make a huge difference in the early days of parenthood. We also need to build a network of other parents who get it, who have been there or are in it now, going through it just like you. Whether via online support groups, local parent meetups, or just going to the nearby park and meeting others, we need connection with others we can have honest conversations with. We need our village, our community, our support system, for so many things when we have a baby. And this does not just mean people to help us with taking care of the baby or our home, but also people who help us take care of ourselves—people who validate our feelings, encourage us and cheerlead for us, and are there to listen when we have a bad day or want to run away and forget the whole being-a-parent thing.

Social media can be a curse in many ways when we compare ourselves to others, but it also can be a place to turn to find our community. When my first daughter was born, I joined a new parents support group, which met weekly for six weeks and discussed different new parenting topics. All of the other birth parents in the group had babies around the same age as my baby, so we were going through the early phase of parenthood together. There were ten people in the group, and two of them became my good friends. Even though they have since moved out of New York City, I can still call or text about anything years later and know I would get an understanding response.

Just as there are rituals in certain cultures around caring for the birth parent in the immediate postpartum period, there are rituals in some cultures that help to establish community. In Iceland, parents take the new baby for a walk, where they introduce their new addition and are met with support and offers to help from the neighborhood. In Australia, the birth parent is brought into a circle of mothers, and everyone relays their own stories of giving birth and bringing home their new babies. The new parent feels validated in their own experience and gains advice about how to handle the common struggles of new parenthood.

If our society acknowledged new parenthood for what it is, it would have to acknowledge the importance of caregiving and the necessity of putting resources and support in place to actually accomplish the tasks associated with caring for a child while also returning to work so that we can afford to live in this country. So how do we create community in a society that prides individuality, self-sufficiency, and self-sacrifice? How do we create community in a society that does not acknowledge that having a baby is one of the most life-altering, difficult, and time-consuming endeavors anyone can undertake?

We start to change the system by creating communities and talking about how freaking hard it is. We validate each other. We share tips and resources we have found to make our lives a little easier. We offer to take turns watching each other's kids so we can get the necessary things done to keep our lives running and our mental sanity intact. And in our "free time" we start lobbying our legislators to build the infrastructure and social support programs we so desperately need to support young families.

FINDING YOUR COMMUNITY

All of the perinatal therapists and psychiatrists I spoke with unanimously and emphatically stressed the importance of community during the postpartum period. Lucy Hutner, reproductive psychiatrist and cofounder of Phoebe, shared her sentiments with me:

> Giving birth is the very definition of connection. And yet we give birth in a highly individualistic society that does not provide nearly the level of support needed for pregnancy and new parents. When we still lack a federal family leave policy in the United States, that's an indictment of the lack of social infrastructure to support parents. That should be a minimum requirement, and it's not. For many people, it's the first time they realize they cannot do it all alone. When we were starting our company, Phoebe, many of the new parents we interviewed said [that] in order to make their postpartum period better, they needed

a lot more support than they realized. The right kind of affordable, accessible community can be found in lots of places: online (some of the time), through faith-based groups, even in free meetup groups in parks. The best kinds of communities are like teams: they are a group of people going through something similar at a similar time, with the same positive end goal in mind.[1]

There are many inclusive and supportive organizations that work hard to create community for new parents. Phoebe, a mental health and well-being platform for expecting and new parents, is one great place to go to find community. Soulside (https://www.getsoulside .com), another startup, also was founded to create an accessible space to build community during pregnancy and postpartum through pregnancy and postpartum groups. Anna Glezer, another wonderful reproductive psychiatrist, joined the team at Soulside because they "really focus on that key part of social support and community, and I think that's so essential for new parents."[2] Oula, the company where I am currently employed as an obstetrician, also understood the importance of providing community support as a part of its holistic care model. It recently started offering Oula Circles, an eight-week virtual postpartum support group where new parents can bring questions about new parenthood and meet other new parents.

My absolute favorite resource for all things perinatal, as I have mentioned in many other chapters of this book, is Postpartum Support International. It offers free virtual support groups, many of which are specialized to different lived experiences, including groups for Black parents, military families, NICU parents, and queer and trans parents. You can find a full list of its weekly offerings on its website.

OTHER WAYS TO CONNECT

A *New York Times* article titled "Making Friends with Other Parents Is Like Dating" gives this pearl of wisdom about the lonely early days of parenthood: "The isolation of the early weeks and months of parenthood is a finite phase, like teething. As your kids age, making friends will become easier, with more opportunities to connect."[3]

However, even in the early days there are ways to connect with other new parents:

- Mommy and Me classes or activities such as story time at your local library, baby swim, and music classes. Many organizations offer free baby classes for newborns up to six months in the hopes that you'll become a paying customer down the road—take advantage of the opportunity to meet other parents!
- Your local faith-based organizations and centers of worship. Many people find support from those with whom they already share a common bond of spirituality.
- Digital communities such as Facebook and Reddit where you can search for other new parents based on shared interests or experiences.
- Virtual and in-person support groups. Some of my favorite free and paid virtual offerings were mentioned earlier. For in-person support groups, check your local new parents groups (most either have a Facebook page or online blog) to see what groups other members of your community recommend. As I mentioned, I met some of my best mom friends through a local in-person group when I was a new overwhelmed mom struggling to get through the days and nights after the birth of my first baby.
- New parent classes. These classes often cover topics from infant feeding to basic infant care and may be run by a clinical person such as a nurse or a nonclinical person such as a doula. You can find these at your local community centers, through your obstetric and pediatric providers, or even through signing up for a course like infant basic life support.
- App-based communities such as Peanut, which started as a meeting place for moms but now has expanded to provide community and support for women through all life stages. Think of it as a dating site for new parents with lots of content.

This may all seem overwhelming and hard to navigate during the early postpartum period. If you have time to think about it before the baby arrives, you can start finding places that resonate with you and making a list of local resources that interest you. Many support groups are due-date based, so you can connect with other parents who will be welcoming their babies around the same time as you and go through the journey together. A lot of new parents and parents-to-be do not realize how lonely and isolating it can feel spending most of your time at home with your new baby, no matter how excited you are and how much you are looking forward to having time at home to welcome them into your life. Infants can't have adult conversations with you, they demand a lot of attention, and it can be overwhelming to take them out in public with all of their stuff at first. This often leads new parents to stay at home alone, feeling emotions they did not anticipate about the reality of their life with their new roommate.

The more you can prepare for this reality in advance—both with your existing support network as well as the community of other parents you are building—the easier it will be to make sure you are surrounded not just by dirty diapers and pump parts, but with other adult humans to keep you from losing touch with the individual human you are, with the same emotions and needs as your beautiful baby.

CONCLUSION

You've Got This!

"Hey mama! How are you doing?"

"Hey mama! I'm just checking in."

"You've got this, mama!"

The person who sent these texts to me during my transition to becoming a new mom is someone whom I had known for years, though we had never become close, intimate friends. She was a dear "friend of a friend," and we had always met up in groups throughout the years I had known her, never one on one. We had never shared our more vulnerable sides with each other, so I was surprised and deeply touched that she was one of the people who made such an impact on my journey.

I should not have been so surprised. *She was a mom already. She knew.*

I had watched her from the outside through both of her transitions to mom and then to mom of two, and she did it all with grace and style. She made it look so easy to me and I aspired to be like her. But she knew. No matter how easy it looks from the outside, pregnancy and the transition to being a parent is *tough*. I felt the silent connection that we had formed as I was initiated into the community of new parents. I am ever so grateful for her small affirmations and acknowledgments that made me realize I was not alone. Every birth parent, no matter how successful, how "together" they appear, and how perfect their lives may seem at times, needs validation and support.

Professionally, I am a doctor who has had the privilege of being a part of the pregnancy, birth, and postpartum journeys of thousands of birthing people. Personally, I feel more like a hype girl. I spend most of my time supporting others, validating their emotions, and affirming that, yes, having a baby is freaking hard. I am paying it forward now. Because *I've been there.* And *I know.*

Approximately 368,000 babies are born every day throughout the world.[1] Because giving birth is so common, many people, before giving birth or becoming a parent themselves, may take it for granted that it must be easy. After all, why would everyone continue to do it—and often do it over and over again—if it was so hard? The fact is that just because something is a common event does not mean that it is easy. A peer-pressure or societal stigma almost seems to exist around verbalizing the difficult aspects of it. Talking about the difficulties of parenthood will ruin the fantasy, revealing the deep truth that as much as we may plan and prepare, there are many aspects of giving birth and the aftermath over which we have no control. This is a really scary thought.

Society treats the journey of becoming a parent as just a normal part of the life cycle, but for the birthing people who experience the hormonal changes, physical changes, emotional changes, spiritual changes, and new self-identity that comes with this rite of passage, even small acknowledgments and encouragements can make a huge impact. If we admit how hard giving birth and having an infant is, then we must admit that we should do a better job supporting the people going through this massive and strenuous undertaking. If we admit that caring for a tiny human being is one of the hardest jobs someone can ever undertake, then we have to admit that we should respect and uplift those who do the majority of caretaking in the world, which falls disproportionately on women. Instead, maintaining the current social structure and relegating primary caregivers to the invisible world inside the home lets the system continue to exploit them, without monetary value given to this labor and without free and affordable social structures in place to support them. Perhaps we will bring to light how terrible the infrastructure supporting new parents, especially the birthing parents, is in our society. To acknowledge what a terrible job we are doing supporting birthing people and new parents would mean acknowledging that we need to change the system.

So yeah, when it comes down to it, I'm here to tell you having a baby may be the hardest thing you ever do in your life. It may go completely differently than you expect. There may be complications you never anticipated or thought would happen to you. It can be beautiful and brutal and everything in between at the same time. It will test you and force you to grow and become uncomfortable and vulnerable in ways you never could have imagined. It will trigger you and bring up parts of your own childhood, both good and bad. But that doesn't mean you shouldn't do it if being a parent is something you really want to do.

Having a baby (or more than one) may also fill you with joy and love and bring new meaning to your existence on this planet. The truth is that no matter how much of a failure you think you are, how many mistakes you think you make, you are still a competent parent. Parent in the way that you feel is the best for your family and to hell with anyone who tries to guilt or shame you into conforming to their way. When others judge you, they do so because their egos, the place where they measure their own value to society and their sense of self-worth, are tied to external markers of success, such as how well they believe they are parenting. If your way is also valid, they may feel that it diminishes all of the hard work they have put into being a "good" parent. But that is their problem, not yours. Keep doing what feels like the best decision for your own well-being and that of your family. Keep doing you.

On the other hand, when you see another parent doing something different from how you would do it, try your best not to give them looks of disapproval, make comments, give unsolicited advice, or generally judge or shame them so that you feel superior or better than them in some way. I have been out many times with my two kids when one or both are melting down. I always appreciate the knowing looks of solidarity I get from other moms. Because we've all been there. I've also been on the playground with my baby and had someone else tell me my baby is not dressed appropriately for the weather and received disapproving looks for pulling out the formula to give to my crying baby. As if I haven't already dealt with the internal guilt and shame around not exclusively breastfeeding. No one needs that kind of judgment from others as well.

Always keep in mind that we do not know someone else's history. What they have gone through, what parts of their journey were choices for a certain reason or because they didn't have a better option. Just trust that they are doing what is best for them and their family. When I see a mom struggling to get her stroller up the steps of the train station, I offer to help when I can. When I see someone trying to get through their grocery shopping with a toddler screaming for any of the million reasons toddlers scream, I give her a smile that says, "I get it." Because I've been there, as well, overwhelmed and trying to do it all as best as I can.

Our best is all we can do; it's all any of us do. And sometimes, honestly, I don't even do my best because I am burned out or need some time for myself. And that's okay as well. Good enough is just that: it's damn sure good enough. So to get off of my soapbox and end this labor of love that comes directly from the heart and soul of someone who never wants you to feel like a failure or a bad parent because of the surprising, unexpected aspects of your journey—the parts that don't align with how society tells us it should be—I want you to know that you are never alone. I guarantee many of us have been there before. And we've made it through to the other side. Through our own tenacity and with lots of hard work and often uncomfortable personal growth. With the help and love of our support network and the compassion and solidarity of strangers. It may seem like it will never get easier, but it does. It gets better. Just like all of us who have come before, no matter what the day ahead brings, just remember: *you've got this.*

ACKNOWLEDGMENTS

Thank you to all of my incredible patients who have trusted me during the most vulnerable parts of their lives. For your courage in telling your stories, even the parts that make you feel shame, guilt, and fear for the future. Your bravery and strength when things don't go as planned, when you face unspeakable tragedies that make me wonder how you have the fortitude to get up another day and go on when I imagine I myself would be a broken shell of a human. I am perpetually in awe and humbled. You are all my guides and my teachers, and this book is as much yours as it is mine.

Thank you to the two little humans, Cahya and Lyla, who transformed my world, turning it upside down and inside out in all of the best ways. Without you, I wouldn't have written this book.

Shaloub, even though our paths have diverged, our girls will always undoubtedly be the best thing either of us has ever put out into the world. Thank you for being such a wonderful coparent on this incredible journey with them.

Sara, thank you for loving every part of me and supporting me in such a way that even during the most emotionally intense year of my life I was able to write this book. Creativity comes from abundance, and you, *mon coeur*, have given me so much love that it has overflowed onto the pages of this book.

Lauren, thank you for holding my hand through all of the struggles that shaped me and led to this book. And for teaching me to be a woman who has the audacity to believe in herself and her mission so much that she convinces others to believe as well.

My two moms, I could not fully appreciate what motherhood meant until Cahya came into this world. Although we all have very different stories as mothers, I see you both in a new light and am so grateful I was blessed with two loving, supportive, and ever-present moms. Thank you for always being there.

Christen Karniski, Joanna Wattenberg, Erin McGarvey, and the team at Rowman & Littlefield, thank you for your support and guidance. Writing and publishing this book is a dream many years in the making, and I feel so honored that you believe in me and the message of this book enough to bring it to life and share it with the world.

Lynnette Novack and the team at the Seymour Agency, thank you for taking a chance on me as a first-time author. You saw the importance of this topic and were my champion, passionately pitching my book until you were confident it was in the hands of the right people. May this be the first of many journeys together.

Ariel Curry, you calmly and gently encouraged and guided me, giving structure and feedback but never taking away my voice. You were the perfect writing coach for me and this book and I am so grateful that Christen recommended we connect. Your magical touch shaped this book, making it something so much more than I ever could have accomplished without you. May our paths meet again.

Tiffany Fung and the team at Biotic Artlab, thank you for your beautiful illustrations that have helped capture some of the parts of giving birth that are often so difficult to grasp and for doing so in such an inclusive and nuanced way. It was such an honor to work with you.

Tawny Lara, you helped me take my passionate ideas and turn them into a book proposal, which was like learning a new language in the span of a few months. Thank you for supporting and guiding me as I hustled to get the proposal completed and submitted before Lyla's birth. I couldn't have done it without your incredible energy and cheerleading!

Anne Lipton, you had the key that unlocked the mysterious entry to finding an agent. I never knew it required more than just a great proposal to get agents to actually open your emails until you came along. Without you, I would have never made it past the entry point, and I thank you so much for your keen advice.

Ashton Renshaw, you helped me get through the final phase, the part I was dreading the most. Thank you so much for taking care of all of the important details prior to submission. You have saved this not-so-tech-savvy, early millennial author many moments of frustration and anxiety!

To all of my colleagues who contributed to this book both directly and indirectly, you are the healers and the givers of the world. You kindly and gently hold space for all of the people you work with every day and for everyone who reads your words in this text. I thank you for all you do to make pregnancy and new parenthood a little bit easier and for sharing your wisdom in this book—your words will be a salve to many.

And to all of my friends and the other moms I have met along the way who have given me the community I needed during the hardest parts of my journey into parenthood. Your validation and support mean more than I can ever say. It takes a village and I am grateful for every single one of you who has been a part of mine.

APPENDIX A

Setting Up Your Environment for Success

Vaishnavi Tallury, MA, OTR/L, PMH-C

1. If keeping your newborn in your room, put the bassinet on your partner's side of the room so they can pick up and change the baby before bringing baby to you for feeding (or feeding baby themselves).
2. Ensure you have safe spaces to put baby for naps during the day in multiple locations around your home, such as having a bassinet on the main floor of your house to avoid going up and down stairs. This is especially important if you have a C-section.
3. Set up multiple changing stations on each floor of your home if you live in a multilevel house.

   * Each changing station should have diapers, wipes, diaper rash ointment, changes of clothes for baby, and change of clothes for you. Optional: keep extra bibs, baby blankets, changing pads, and burp clothes in this location to keep everything in one place.
   * Have your partner check and restock these stations every couple of days to ensure you have what you need during the day.

4. Keep all items at waist or hip level to minimize reaching and bending when changing your baby.
5. Avoid hunching over to change baby, pick up baby, or feed baby. Bend with your knees!
6. Prevent De Quervain's tenosynovitis ("mommy's thumb") by keeping your thumbs next to your palms and support baby with one hand under their bottom and one hand on their neck/back. Do not make an *L* shape with your hands to scoop baby under their armpits, because this can strain your wrists and thumbs.

7. Keep multiple pillows and folding footstools nearby for ergonomic support when feeding.

   * Aim to keep your neck and shoulders in a neutral position. Avoid hiking up your shoulder toward your ear when you support baby in your arms.
   * Your back should be supported by pillows or cushions so that you are sitting upright or leaning slightly back in a relaxed position and not hunched over.
   * Keep your hips flexed and knees bent at 90 degrees, using a footstool if needed. Bring baby to you, do not lean forward to feed baby!

8. Keep high-protein snacks and a large water bottle with a straw near your feeding stations so you can eat and drink while baby does.
9. Cue up TV shows, podcasts, or audiobooks to entertain you and help you relax. Limit scrolling the internet and social media as much as you can.
10. Put receiving blankets/baby blankets on every surface you put your baby down on. This will reduce your baby coming into contact with allergens (body fluids, pet hair, dust, etc.). It also protects your bedding, furniture, and rugs from baby messes and makes cleanup much easier!
11. Keep multiple changing pads/diaper bags ready by the door or in your stroller or car so that you aren't scrambling to find diapers and wipes when you leave the house. Put a changing pad, a pack of wipes, a few diapers, and a change of clothes in a wet bag by the door for easy grabbing!

APPENDIX B

Postpartum Emotions Chart

Use this chart to track whether you are impacted by emotional concerns postpartum.

Not impacted	Baby blues	Postpartum depression	Postpartum anxiety
Tears of joy or frustration on occasion.	Random **tears** (even for a toilet paper ad) that come out of nowhere.	**Tearfulness** that may or may not have a direct cause.	**Tears** around thoughts that might be scary.
Sleep deprived but able to nap during the day. No issues falling or staying asleep.	Learning to **sleep** when the baby sleeps. Getting used to sleep/wake cycle that you aren't used to.	**Sleep** is interrupted in one of two ways: difficulty rousing oneself (consistently) or unable to fall and stay asleep.	Difficulties falling and staying **asleep**. Not able to sleep due to racing thoughts.
Your **mind** might feel clumsy at times and forgetful, but you are able to carry on a conversation (unless the baby interrupts).	Your **mind** feels a little foggy and it might be hard to focus.	Your **mind** feels full and it can be hard to express yourself. You might feel forgetful or distracted. Carrying on a conversation can be difficult, and not because of the baby.	Your **mind** is racing and it is hard to slow it down.
You seldom **worry** about things that are new for you.	You **worry** a little and sometimes check in with others and sometimes keep it to yourself.	You feel too sad or angry to **worry**.	You **worry** continually and some of your worries might scare you. You are afraid to tell others about *all* of your worries, though you might share some.

(continued)

Not impacted	Baby blues	Postpartum depression	Postpartum anxiety
The **changes** in your life are exciting and make you look forward to the future.	The **changes** in your life are temporarily overwhelming, but you are able to adjust with a little practice.	The **changes** in your life are completely overwhelming, and you are having difficulty adjusting to them.	The **changes** in your life cause you perpetual worry as you struggle to make sense of them.
Bonding with your baby isn't something that you spend time thinking about, as you do so by caring for your baby.	**Bonding** with your baby is initially awkward, but with practice, you adjust.	**Bonding** with your baby is hard, because you feel detached from your baby and attending to its needs.	**Bonding** with your baby is something that you are thinking a lot about: Are you doing it right? Is your baby attached enough?
After a few weeks, you relish your new routine as your "new normal."	**After a few weeks**, you get the hang of things and start to feel more like yourself.	**After a few weeks**, you feel just as bad, if not worse.	**After a few weeks**, the worrying persists.

Source: Created by Dr. Julie Bindeman, Integrative Therapy of Greater Washington (drbindeman@gmail.com).

NOTES

CHAPTER ONE

1. Kelsey L. Power, PhD, licensed clinical psychologist and reproductive mental health specialist, www.kelseypowerphd.com.

CHAPTER TWO

1. Emanuel A. Friedman, "The Graphic Analysis of Labor," *American Journal of Obstetrics and Gynecology* 68, no. 6 (1954): 1568–75, https://doi.org/10.1016/0002-9378(54)90311-7.

2. Saonjie F. Hamilton, CNM, https://oulahealth.com/.

CHAPTER THREE

1. *Inside Edition*, "Is This Salad the Secret to Inducing Labor?" YouTube, June 9, 2023, https://www.youtube.com/watch?v=FwHo8Xjwg5M.

2. William A. Grobman, Madeline M. Rice, Uma M. Reddy, Alan T. N. Tita, Robert M. Silver, Gail Mallett et al. "Labor Induction Versus Expectant Management in Low-Risk Nulliparous Women," *New England Journal of Medicine* 379, no. 6 (2018): 513–23, https://doi.org/10.1056/nejmoa1800566.

3. Saonjie F. Hamilton, CNM, https://oulahealth.com/.

4. "Bishop Score Calculator," Perinatology.com, 2014, https://perinatology.com/calculators/Bishop%20Score%20Calculator.htm.

CHAPTER FIVE

1. Joyce A. Martin, Brady E. Hamilton, Michelle J. K. Osterman, and Anne K. Driscoll, "Births: Final Data for 2019," *National Vital Statistics Reports* 70, no. 2 (2021): https://dx.doi.org/10.15620/cdc:100472.

2. Nathalie Roos, Lena Sahlin, Gunvor Ekman-Ordeberg, Helle Kieler, and Olof Stephansson, "Maternal Risk Factors for Postterm Pregnancy and Cesarean Delivery Following Labor Induction," *Acta Obstetricia Et Gynecologica Scandinavica* 89, no. 8 (2010): 1003–10, https://doi.org/10.3109/0001 6349.2010.500009.

CHAPTER SEVEN

1. Fed Is Best Foundation, "Our Mission: Safe Breastfeeding and Bottle-feeding Support," May 27, 2024, https://fedisbest.org/.

2. Vaishnavi Tallury, MA, OTR/L, PMH-C, www.sevenmothersot.com.

CHAPTER NINE

1. "Baby Blues after Pregnancy," March of Dimes, May 2021, https://www.marchofdimes.org/find-support/topics/postpartum/baby-blues-after-pregnancy#:~:text=Baby%20blues%20are%20feelings%20of,blame%20for%20how%20you%20feel.

2. See appendix B.

3. Christie Lancaster Palladino, Vijay Singh, Jacquelyn Campbell, Heather Flynn, and Katherine Gold, "Homicide and Suicide during the Perinatal Period: Findings from the National Violent Death Reporting System," *Obstetrics & Gynecology* 118, no. 5 (November 2011): 1056–63, https://doi.org/10.1097/AOG.0b013e31823294da.

4. World Health Organization, "Mental Health and COVID-19: Early Evidence of the Pandemic's Impact: Scientific Brief, 2 March 2022," scientific brief, March 2, 2022, https://www.who.int/publications/i/item/WHO-2019-nCoV-Sci_Brief-Mental_health-2022.1.

5. Qianqian Chen, Wenjie Li, Juan Xiong, and Xujuan Zheng, "Prevalence and Risk Factors Associated with Postpartum Depression during the COVID-19 Pandemic: A Literature Review and Meta-Analysis," *International Journal of Environmental Research and Public Health/International Journal of Environmental Research and Public Health* 19, no. 4 (2022): 2219, https://doi.org/10.3390/ijerph19042219.

6. Child Welfare Information Gateway, "Child Welfare Practice to Address Racial Disproportionality and Disparity," *Bulletins for Professionals*, April 2021, https://cwig-prod-prod-drupal-s3fs-us-east-1.s3.amazonaws.com/public/documents/racial_disproportionality.pdf.

7. Mia Hemstad, "Black Women, Birthing People, and Maternal Mental Health Fact Sheet," Maternal Mental Health Leadership Alliance, April 16,

2024, https://www.mmhla.org/articles/black-women-birthing-people-mothers-and-maternal-mental-health-fact-sheet.

8. Susannah Cahalan, "Is Fear the Last Taboo of Motherhood?" *New York Times*, April 7, 2020, https://www.nytimes.com/2020/04/07/books/review/ordinary-insanity-fear-motherhood-sarah-menkedick.html.

9. Sarah Menkedick, *Ordinary Insanity* (New York: Penguin Random House, 2020).

10. Lisa Tremayne, RN, PMH-C, https://www.rwjbh.org/our-locations/out patient-rehab-center/center-for-perinatal-mood-and-anxiety-disorders-/.

11. Lucy A. Hutner, MD, New York City–based reproductive psychiatrist and cofounder of Phoebe, Inc., www.lucyhutnermd.com.

12. Anna Glezer, MD, reproductive and integrative psychiatrist, https://anna glezermd.com/.

13. Cheryl Tatano Beck, Sue Watson, and Robert K. Gable, "Traumatic Child-birth and Its Aftermath: Is There Anything Positive?" *The Journal of Perinatal Education* 27, no. (32018): 175–84, https://doi.org/10.1891/1058-1243.27.3.175.

14. Jaz Robbins, PsyD, BCHN, psychologist and nutritionist, https://www.drjazrobbins.com/.

15. Dr. Julie Bindeman, PsyD, reproductive psychologist, www.GreaterWash ingtonTherapy.com.

16. Kelsey L. Power, PhD, licensed clinical psychologist and reproductive mental health specialist, www.kelseypowerphd.com.

CHAPTER TEN

1. Baby-Friendly USA, *Interim Guidelines and Evaluation Criteria for Facilities Seeking Baby-Friendly Designation* (Albany, NY: Baby-Friendly USA, 2019), https://www.babyfriendlyusa.org/wp-content/uploads/2019/12/US-Interim-GEC_191107_CLEAN.pdf.

2. The US Department of Health and Human Services, Office of Disease Prevention and Health Promotion, Healthy People 2020 guidelines have been updated and are available at https://www.healthypeople.gov/2020.

3. Christie del Castillo-Hegyi, MD, emergency physician, cofounder of the Fed Is Best Foundation, https://fedisbest.org.

4. M. Neifert, "Prevention of Breastfeeding Tragedies," *Pediatric Clinics of North America* 48, no. 2 (2001): 273–97, https://doi.org/10.1016/s0031-3955 (08)70026-9.

5. Emily Oster, *Cribsheet* (New York: Penguin, 2019), https://parentdata .org/wp-content/uploads/2023/12/9e9cc18a-fd95-4526-a382-7603cb45c12a .pdf; Emily Oster, "Breast Is Best? Breast Is Better? Breast Is about the Same?" ParentData, April 29, 2024, https://parentdata.org/breast-is-best-breast-is -better-breast-is-about-the-same/.

6. Centers for Disease Control and Prevention, Division of Nutrition, Physical Activity, and Obesity, "Breastfeeding Report Card United States, 2020," 2020, https://www.cdc.gov/breastfeeding/pdf/2020-breastfeeding-report-card -h.pdf.

7. Alia M. Heise and Diane Wiessinger, "Dysphoric Milk Ejection Reflex: A Case Report," *International Breastfeeding Journal* 6, no. 6 (2011), https://doi .org/10.1186/1746-4358-6-6.

8. "Newt—Newborn Weight Tool," Newt, November 29, 2016, https://new bornweight.org/.

9. Lynette Hafken, MA, IBCLC, lactation and infant feeding consultant, https://rockvillelactation.com.

10. S. E. Daly, R. A. Owens, and P. E. Hartmann, "The Short-Term Synthesis and Infant-Regulated Removal of Milk in Lactating Women," *Experimental Physiology* 78, no. 2 (1993): 209–20, https://doi.org/10.1113/expphysiol.1993 .sp003681; J. C. Kent, L. R. Mitoulas, M. D. Cregan, D. T. Ramsay, D. A. Doherty, and P. E. Hartmann, "Volume and Frequency of Breastfeedings and Fat Content of Breast Milk throughout the Day," *Pediatrics*, 117, no. 3 (2006): e387-95, https://doi.org/10.1542/peds.2005-1417.

CHAPTER ELEVEN

1. Ronit Sukenick, PT, DPT, PRPC, pelvic floor physical therapy specialist, https://www.foundations-pt.com.

2. Joanie Johnson, pre- and postnatal corrective exercise specialist, diastasis and core consultant, https://www.youtube.com/@corrective.exercise.workouts, www.transformation-nation.com.

3. Brianna Houston, pregnancy and postpartum strength expert, longevity athleticism coach, https://www.andbeyondtraining.com/.

4. Jaz Robbins, PsyD, BCHN, psychologist and nutritionist, https://www .drjazrobbins.com/.

CHAPTER TWELVE

1. Catharine McDonald, MS, NCC, LPC, PMH-C, perinatal sex therapist and reproductive mental health therapist and owner and clinical director of Growing Well Counseling, https://www.growingwellcounseling.com.

2. Jaz Robbins, PsyD, BCHN, psychologist and nutritionist, https://www
.drjazrobbins.com/.

3. Andrew Wheeler, board-certified pastoral counselor, and Elizabeth
Wheeler, licensed clinical pastor, PMH-C, https://www.wheelerandwheeler
counseling.com/.

CHAPTER THIRTEEN

1. Shari Thurer, *The Myths of Motherhood: How Culture Reinvents the Good
Mother* (New York: Penguin, 1995), xii.

CHAPTER FOURTEEN

1. Margaret Swarbrick, "A Wellness Approach," *Psychiatric Rehabilitation
Journal* 29, no. 4 (2006): 311–14, https://doi.org/10.2975/29.2006.311.314.

2. Pooja Lakshmin, *Real Self-Care (Crystals, Cleanses, and Bubble Baths Not
Included)* (New York: Penguin Life, 2023).

3. Tracy Torelli, therapist, educator, and women's mental health specialist,
www.claritytherapycny.com.

4. Andrew Wheeler, board-certified pastoral counselor, and Elizabeth
Wheeler, licensed clinical pastor, PMH-C, https://www.wheelerandwheeler
counseling.com/.

CHAPTER FIFTEEN

1. Lucy A. Hutner, MD, New York City–based reproductive psychiatrist and
cofounder of Phoebe, Inc., www.lucyhutnermd.com.

2. Anna Glezer, MD, reproductive and integrative psychiatrist, https://anna
glezermd.com/.

3. "Making Friends with Other Parents Is Like Dating," *New York Times*,
April 15, 2020, https://www.nytimes.com/article/making-parent-friends-guide
.html.

CONCLUSION

1. "Births per Year," Our World in Data, 2024, https://ourworldindata.org
/grapher/number-of-births-per-year.

BIBLIOGRAPHY

"Baby Blues after Pregnancy." March of Dimes. May 2021. https://
www.marchofdimes.org/find-support/topics/postpartum/baby-blues
-after-pregnancy.

Baby-Friendly USA. *Interim Guidelines and Evaluation Criteria for Facilities
Seeking Baby-Friendly Designation.* Albany, NY: Baby-Friendly USA, 2019.
https://www.babyfriendlyusa.org/wp-content/uploads/2019/12/US
-Interim-GEC_191107_CLEAN.pdf.

"Births per Year." Our World in Data. 2024. https://ourworldindata.org
/grapher/number-of-births-per-year.

"Bishop Score Calculator." Perinatology.com. 2014. https://perinatology
.com/calculators/Bishop%20Score%20Calculator.htm.

Cahalan, Susannah. "Is Fear the Last Taboo of Motherhood?" *New York
Times,* April 7, 2020. https://www.nytimes.com/2020/04/07/books/
review/ordinary-insanity-fear-motherhood-sarah-menkedick.html.

Centers for Disease Control and Prevention, Division of Nutrition, Physical
Activity, and Obesity. "Breastfeeding Report Card United States, 2020."
2020. https://www.cdc.gov/breastfeeding/pdf/2020-breastfeeding-report
-card-h.pdf.

Friedman, Emanuel A. "The Graphic Analysis of Labor." *American Journal
of Obstetrics and Gynecology* 68, no. 6 (1954): 1568–75. https://doi.org
/10.1016/0002-9378(54)90311-7.

Heise, Alia M., and Diane Wiessinger. "Dysphoric Milk Ejection Reflex: A
Case Report." *International Breastfeeding Journal* 6, no. 6 (2011): https://
doi.org/10.1186/1746-4358-6-6.

"Making Friends with Other Parents Is Like Dating," *New York Times,* April
15, 2020. https://www.nytimes.com/article/making-parent-friends-guide
.html.

Martin, Joyce A., Brady E. Hamilton, Michelle J. K. Osterman, and Anne K.
Driscoll. "Births: Final Data for 2019." *National Vital Statistics Reports* 70,
no. 2 (2021): https://dx.doi.org/10.15620/cdc:100472.

Neifert, M. "Prevention of Breastfeeding Tragedies." *Pediatric Clinics of North America* 48, no. 2 (2001): 273–97, https://doi.org/10.1016/s0031-3955(08)70026-9.

"Newt—Newborn Weight Loss Tool." Newt. November 29, 2016. https://newbornweight.org/.

Menkedick, Sarah. *Ordinary Insanity*. New York: Penguin Random House, 2020.

Oster, Emily. "Breast Is Best? Breast Is Better? Breast Is about the Same?" ParentData, April 29, 2024. https://parentdata.org/breast-is-best-breast-is-better-breast-is-about-the-same/.

Palladino, Christie Lancaster, Vijay Singh, Jacquelyn Campbell, Heather Flynn, and Katherine Gold. "Homicide and Suicide during the Perinatal Period: Findings from the National Violent Death Reporting System." *Obstetrics & Gynecology* 118, no. 5 (November 2011): 1056–63, https://doi.org/10.1097/AOG.0b013e31823294da.

Swarbrick, Margaret. "A Wellness Approach." *Psychiatric Rehabilitation Journal* 29, no. 4 (2006): 311–14, https://doi.org/10.2975/29.2006.311.314.

RESOURCES

The following includes recommended resources from experts I trust.

PREGNANCY

Pregnancy and postpartum compression shorts and postpartum compression shorts: https://srchealth.com
Serola sacroiliac belt: https://www.serola.net
V2 supporter for vulvar varicosities: https://itsyoubabe.com/product/v2-supporter/
Physio ball (65 cm is usually a good size for most people): https://www.performancehealth.com/theraband-standard-exercise-balls
Expecting Better by Emily Oster
Like a Mother: A Feminist Journey through the Science and Culture of Pregnancy by Angela Garbes
The Birth of a Mother by Daniel Stern
The Motherhood Center: https://themotherhoodcenter.com/
For neurodiverse mothers: http://www.strugglecare.com/

LACTATION AND FEEDING

Lynnette Hafken, MA, IBCLC, lactation and infant feeding consultant: https://rockvillelactation.com
Christie del Castillo-Hegyi, MD, emergency physician, cofounder of the Fed Is Best Foundation: Fedisbestbook.org
Breastfeeding support group: https://www.facebook.com/groups/breastfeedingconfidential
La Leche League: https://llli.org/
World Health Organization: https://www.who.int/health-topics/breastfeeding#tab=tab_1

Proper storage of breast milk: https://www.cdc.gov/breastfeeding/
recommendations/handling_breastmilk.htm

SEX AND INTIMACY

OMGYES (www.omgyes.com): A great place to find guidance
around self-pleasure both in technique and communication,
tasteful instructional writing, and videos with realistic portrayals
of different bodies exploring pleasure.

Bedsider (www.bedsider.org): The self-described "online birth control support network" has some great sex-positive, body-positive
articles, excellent information about contraception choices, and
details regarding how to access reproductive healthcare including
telemedicine.

Clue (www.helloclue.com): Not only a secure cycle tracker, but this
app has a brilliant encyclopedia full of factual information on
all things reproduction related including fertility, pregnancy, and
loss—including specific scenarios like menstrual cycles after a
miscarriage. It often offers a discount code for their paid app
services!

The Gottman Card Decks app (https://www.gottman.com/couples
/apps/): It can be such a great resource for couples to use for
building conversation and connection in daily life, date nights,
sex life, as well as preparing for baby.

Good Clean Love vaginal moisturizer with hyaluronic acid: https://
goodcleanlove.com/products/bionourish®-ultra-moisturizing
-vaginal-gel-with-hyaluronic-acid-assortment?variant=42220
336218296

BIRTH/REPRODUCTIVE TRAUMA

Australasian Birth Trauma Association: https://birthtrauma.org.au/
Unfold Your Wings: https://unfoldyourwings.co.uk/
Bereavement or PAIL (pregnancy and infant loss doula): https://
evidencebasedbirth.com/grief-and-healing-through-pregnancy
-and-infant-loss-with-full-spectrum-d oula-rose-rankin/

MENTAL HEALTH

The Center for Women's Mental Health: http://www.womensmental
health.org/
Postpartum Support International: https://www.postpartum.net/

POSTPARTUM SUPPORT

Postpartum Support International: https://www.postpartum.net/get
-help/loss-grief-in-pregnancy-postpartum/
For the new mother: 4th Trimester Project (https://www.newmom
health.com/help/)
Meal train: https://fedandfit.com/meal-train-how-to/
The First Forty Days: The Essential Art of Nourishing the New Mother
by Heng Ou
Fair Play by Eve Rodsky
Dr. Becky Kennedy: Good Inside (https://www.goodinside.com)
Oula Circles (https://oulahealth.com/): An eight-week virtual post-
partum support group and place to bring any of your questions
about new parenthood and to meet other new parents.
Practice Brave Podcast: https://open.spotify.com/show/1P1X8ylAy
GPxc3dtzMBzGE?si=5bce31152bae4ca9
Exercise cheat sheets for pregnancy and for the first six weeks post-
partum: https://www.briannabattles.com/resources/
*Real Self-Care: A Transformative Program for Redefining Wellness (Crys-
tals, Cleanses, and Bubble Baths Not Included)* by Pooja Lackshmin
Set Boundaries, Find Peace: A Guide to Reclaiming Yourself by Nedra
Glover Tawwab

HEALING POSTPARTUM

Serenity Pelvic Wand: www.cmtmedical.com/product/serenity-tmt
-pelvic-floor-massage-tool-vaginal/
Squatty Potty: www.squattypotty.com
Silicone strips for C-section scars: https://marena.com/products/
silicone-scar-strip

The Lotus Method Newsletter: https://9ec29b91-bd8b-48fa-a7b8
-a4c0148bb6b6.myflodesk.com/h8cr8mf5yj

FREE RESOURCES RECOMMENDED BY THE AUTHOR

For NICU parents: https://handtohold.org/nicu-family-support/nicu
-support-groups/

Virtual peer support and parenting classes: https://www.justbirth
space.org/en/communityconnect

Support for black birthing people: https://www.shematters.health/
online-community

Curated content and meditations: https://expectful.com

Community and inspirational content: https://www.mycheckonmom
.com/ and www.catrionahippman.com/research-video

Pregnancy loss support: https://www.pregnancyloss.org/

Ending a wanted pregnancy: https://endingawantedpregnancy.com/

LGBTQ resources: https://www.perinatalnyc.com/services/#queer
and https://familyequality.org/neighborhood/

INDEX

ABOUT THE AUTHOR

Dr. Jessica Vernon, MD, PMH-C, is a board-certified OB/GYN who has cared for and supported thousands of people throughout their reproductive journeys over the past fifteen years. She is the clinical director of product as well as an associate medical director at Oula, a midwifery-based women's health startup in New York City. As a mom of two, she brings her lived experience with the transition to parenthood to her work. She has a deep passion for providing holistic, people-centered, culturally humble care and has developed programs to increase access to perinatal mental health care and to improve health equity. She has received professional recognition and has been quoted in the media for both her work and expertise in the field as well as her openness in sharing her own story. *Then Comes Baby* is her first book.